EAT TO RESTORE

The food based path to reverse persistent health problems.

The R.E.S.T.O.R.E. MILA Series: Volume 2

Christopher F. Thoma, DC

307 Longevity

Cody, Wyoming

Part of The R.E.S.T.O.R.E. MILA Series: Volume 2

ISBN: 978-1-971449-03-6

Published by 307 Longevity

1120 Beck Ave. Cody, WY 82414

Third Edition, 2026

Medical Disclaimer

The information provided in this book is for educational and informational purposes only and is not intended as medical advice. It is not a substitute for professional medical advice, diagnosis, or treatment. Always seek the advice of your physician or other qualified health provider with any questions you may have regarding a medical condition. Never disregard professional medical advice or delay in seeking it because of something you have read in this book.

The author and publisher make no representations or warranties of any kind, express or implied, about the completeness, accuracy, reliability, suitability, or availability of the information contained in this book. Any reliance you place on such information is strictly at your own risk.

Table of Contents

Preface

It is with profound gratitude that I share the knowledge contained in these pages. This book represents the culmination of my formal education and four academic degrees, but more importantly, it embodies the wisdom gained from the countless individuals who have honored me with their trust and shared the intimate details of their health journeys.

My patients have been my greatest teachers. Through their struggles, perseverance, and ultimately their healing, they have illuminated the path that conventional medicine often overlooks. For their trust, I am eternally grateful.

The stories you will encounter are drawn from real clinical experiences. However, to honor the privacy of those who have entrusted me with their care, I have created fictional characters based on these real individuals. The medical conditions, symptoms, and transformations described are authentic representations of patterns I have witnessed repeatedly in clinical practice. The names and personal details have been carefully altered to ensure confidentiality while preserving the essential truth of each healing journey.

While the characters you will meet are not real individuals, the science behind their conditions is rigorous, the mechanisms of their dysfunction are accurate, and the transformations they experience reflect what is genuinely possible when we address the root causes of chronic illness.

This work would not have been possible without my family. To my wife, Jennifer, whose patience and encouragement sustained me through countless late nights: your love made this possible.

To my children, Casper and Sadie, who inspire me to create a healthier world for their generation: you are my greatest motivation.

I am deeply grateful to the many professors who shaped my thinking, the doctors and colleagues who refined these concepts through clinical application, and my dedicated employees who help translate these principles into practical protocols that serve those who need them most.

To those reading these words while struggling with chronic health challenges: the stories in this book, though fictionalized, represent real possibilities for your own healing. Science is sound. The pathway is clear. What remains is the courage to begin.

With deep respect and profound gratitude,

Dr. Christopher

Introduction:

The Food Revolution Your Body Has Been Waiting For

Maria walked into my office carrying a three-inch binder filled with test results, specialist referrals, and medication lists. At 52, an elementary school teacher who once loved her job, she could barely make it through a school day without collapsing on her classroom's reading corner couch during lunch. Her joints ached so severely that opening jar lids had become impossible. The brain fog was so thick that she'd started writing lesson plans in her hand to remember what she was teaching. For fifteen years, she'd collected diagnoses like stamps: irritable bowel syndrome, fibromyalgia, chronic fatigue syndrome, and most recently, 'possible autoimmune condition,' origin unknown.

'I've tried everything,' she said, her voice breaking. 'Every medication makes something else worse. I've done elimination diets, gone gluten-free, tried vegan, keto, paleo. I've spent thousands on supplements that promised to fix me. Nothing works for more than a few weeks. The gastroenterologist says my gut is fine, just 'sensitive.' The rheumatologist says my inflammation markers are 'borderline.' The neurologist says the brain fog is from stress. But I know something is deeply wrong. I just don't know what.'

Maria's story wasn't unique. In fact, it was the third time that week I had heard nearly the same narrative. Different symptoms, same pattern: years of chasing symptoms with medications, temporary relief followed by new problems, specialists who could not connect the dots, and a medical system that had given up on finding root causes. Maria did not need another medication or another restrictive diet. She needed to understand what had broken in her body's fundamental operating system, and more importantly, she needed a systematic way to restore it.

The Hidden Crisis in Modern Health

We are living through an unprecedented health paradox. Despite having more medical knowledge, more sophisticated treatments, and more health information than ever before in human history, we are sicker than we have ever been. Chronic disease affects 60% of American adults [1]. Autoimmune conditions have tripled in the last 50 years [2]. Children are developing 'adult' diseases like Type 2 diabetes and fatty liver disease at alarming rates [3]. Something fundamental has shifted, and it's not our genetics, which change over millennia, not decades.

The shift happened in our food supply, and it happened so gradually that most of us never noticed. Over the past century, and accelerating dramatically in the last 50 years, we have transformed food from nourishment into something our bodies no longer recognize. We've introduced thousands of chemicals our cells have never encountered. We have concentrated sugars to levels that overwhelm our metabolic machinery. We have altered the molecular structure of wheat, corn, and soy through intensive hybridization and genetic modification. We replaced traditional fats with industrial seed oils that disrupt cellular communication. We've created a food environment so foreign to our biology that our bodies are mounting constant defensive responses, treating much of what we eat as foreign invaders.

This isn't just about eating 'healthy' rather than 'unhealthy' foods. Even people who think they're making good choices, who shop at health food stores and read every label, are often consuming foods that trigger systemic inflammation and cellular dysfunction. The granola bar marketed as heart-healthy contains four different forms of sugar and inflammatory seed oils. The gluten-free bread that promised digestive relief has twenty-seven ingredients, including emulsifiers that destroy the gut lining. The plant-based meat alternative designed to save the planet contains soy protein isolates, inflammatory oils, and chemical flavoring agents that stress the liver and disrupt hormones.

Understanding Your Body's Operating System: The MILA Framework

To understand why modern food is making us sick, we need to understand how the body actually maintains health. For decades, medicine has approached the body as a collection of separate systems: cardiovascular, digestive, nervous, immune. When something goes wrong, we target that specific system with specialized treatments. But this compartmentalized approach misses the fundamental truth about human biology: everything is connected through what I call the MILA system.

MILA stands for the Mitochondrial-Immune-Lymphatic Axis, and it represents the three interconnected systems that determine whether your body maintains health or descends into chronic disease. Think of it as your body's operating system, like the software that runs your computer. When this operating system functions properly, your body effortlessly maintains balance, repairs damage, fights off threats, and generates abundant energy. When it's corrupted, everything starts to malfunction, leading to the seemingly unrelated symptoms that characterize modern chronic disease.

The mitochondria are your cellular power plants, generating the energy currency (ATP) that fuels every biological process [4]. But they are far more than just energy producers. Mitochondria are also your body's danger sensors, constantly monitoring the cellular environment for threats. When they detect danger, whether from toxins, infections, or metabolic stress, they shift from energy production mode into defensive mode, a state called the Cell Danger Response [5]. This shift is meant to be temporary, but modern food keeps mitochondria locked in danger mode, leading to chronic fatigue, brain fog, and metabolic dysfunction.

The immune system does more than fight infections; it is your body's Department of Homeland Security, maintaining order and responding to threats. But when constantly activated by inflammatory foods, it becomes dysregulated, attacking healthy tissue (autoimmunity), overreacting to harmless substances (allergies), or becoming exhausted and unable to respond properly (immune suppression) [6]. Modern food, particularly the nine categories we'll explore, keeps the immune system in a state of chronic activation, like a smoke alarm that never stops ringing.

The lymphatic system, perhaps the most overlooked component of health, is your body's drainage and recycling system. It removes cellular waste, filters toxins, and maintains fluid balance [7]. When lymphatic flow becomes stagnant, toxins accumulate, tissues become swollen and painful, and the entire terrain of the body becomes polluted. Modern inflammatory foods, combined with sedentary lifestyle, cause lymphatic congestion that turns your internal environment into a toxic swamp where disease thrives.

These three systems don't operate independently: they're in constant communication. When mitochondria detect danger, they signal the immune system to activate. The activated immune system produces inflammatory compounds that further stress mitochondria. Both systems dump their waste into the lymphatic system, which becomes overwhelmed and backs up, creating more inflammation and mitochondrial stress. It's a vicious cycle that modern food perpetuates with every meal.

The R.E.S.T.O.R.E. Protocol: A Systematic Approach to Healing

Understanding the problem is only the first step. The real question is: how do we fix it? This is where most approaches fail. They either try to suppress symptoms with medications, which often make the underlying dysfunction worse, or they attempt random interventions without a systematic plan. Throwing supplements at the problem, trying the latest fad diet, or doing intensive detoxes without proper preparation usually backfires, sometimes spectacularly.

The R.E.S.T.O.R.E. protocol represents a systematic, sequential approach to healing that works with your body's biology rather than against it. Each step builds on the previous one, and the order matters tremendously. Trying to skip ahead or do everything at once is like trying to rebuild a house while it's on fire; you have to put out the fire first.

Reveal - The first step is a comprehensive assessment to understand your unique dysfunction pattern. You must ask the right questions; this is done with the RESTORE MILA Dynamic Intake and the proper testing. This is not about generic blood work that comes back 'normal' despite how terrible you feel. It's about specialized testing that reveals mitochondrial function, immune activation patterns, toxic burden, and nutritional deficiencies at the cellular level. Without proper assessment, you are guessing, and guessing with your health is expensive and dangerous.

Eliminate - This is where the dietary intervention begins, removing the foods that perpetuate MILA dysfunction. We are not talking about a temporary diet or a 30-day cleanse. We're talking about eliminating specific categories of foods that your body treats as toxins. I call these the Toxic Nine, and they're hiding in nearly everything we eat. This elimination isn't about deprivation; it's about removing the obstacles to healing so your body can do what it is designed to do: heal itself. This is also where we focus on helping the lymphatic system eliminate those harmful things we have already put into our bodies.

Strengthen - Once we have stopped the damage, we begin rebuilding balance in our immune system. This means strengthening digestive function, supporting liver detoxification pathways, and beginning to restore proper immune function. Think of it as reinforcing the foundation before rebuilding the house. Many people try to skip this step and jump straight to killing infections or overstimulating the immune system, which is like trying to clean a house while the roof is caving in.

Turbocharge - With foundations strong, we can now optimize cellular energy production. This involves targeted mitochondrial support, hormone optimization, and metabolic restoration. This is where energy begins returning, brain fog lifts, and people start feeling like themselves again. But it only works if we have properly prepared the terrain; otherwise, we're just reviewing a broken engine.

Optimize - Now we fine-tune the system, addressing individual weaknesses and maximizing strengths. This involves targeted supplementation for specific deficiencies, returning the natural circadian rhythms and cortisol patterns, and supporting glymphatic drainage. This is the point we see neurotransmitters begin to work as intended, brain fog lift and clear thought and memory come back to normal. It's personalized medicine at its finest but built on the solid foundation of the previous steps.

Repair - This phase focuses on tissue regeneration. This is where we rebuild damaged tissues restore healthy patterns, that you may have thought would never be possible again.

Everlasting Health - The final phase transitions from active treatment to maintenance and longevity. Ongoing lifestyle practices, seasonal drainage resets, and continued MILA awareness sustain long-term resilience and prevent relapses. For those who want to go beyond restoration to optimization, this phase focuses on performance enhancement, longevity protocols, and achieving peak human potential. But it is only possible after we've restored basic function; you cannot optimize a broken system.

The Toxic Nine: Foods That Are Breaking Your Biology

At the heart of the R.E.S.T.O.R.E. protocol's dietary intervention is the elimination of what I call the Toxic Nine, nine categories of foods that drive MILA dysfunction. These are not foods your great-grandparents would recognize, even though some carry familiar names. Through processing, genetic modification, chemical treatment, and industrial production methods, we've transformed these foods into substances that trigger systemic inflammation, disrupt cellular communication, and keep the body locked in a state of chronic stress.

The Toxic Nine are:

1. Sugar in all forms - Not just table sugar, but the 61 different names food manufacturers use to hide it. The average American consumes 150-170 pounds of sugar per year, compared to 5 pounds in 1900 [8]. This 3,000% increase has overwhelmed our metabolic machinery, leading to mitochondrial dysfunction, immune dysregulation, and systemic inflammation.

2. Modern wheat and gluten - Today's wheat bears little resemblance to ancestral varieties. Through intensive hybridization, we've created dwarf wheat with 50% more gluten and novel proteins that trigger zonulin release, opening the tight junctions in the gut lining [9]. This is not just about celiac disease; non-celiac gluten sensitivity affects up to 13% of the population [10].

3. Corn (especially GMO and HFCS) - 92% of US corn is genetically modified to produce its own pesticide or resist herbicides [11]. High fructose corn syrup, found in every processed food, drives fatty liver disease and metabolic dysfunction. Even organic corn products can trigger inflammation in sensitive individuals.

4. Unfermented soy - 94% of US soy is genetically modified and heavily contaminated with glyphosate [11]. Soy protein isolates, found in everything from protein bars to meat alternatives, contain phytoestrogens that disrupt hormones and anti-nutrients that block mineral absorption.

5. Conventional dairy - Modern dairy from A1 casein cows produces BCM-7, an opioid peptide that triggers inflammation and digestive issues [12]. Add in lactose intolerance affecting 65-70% of the global population, plus hormones, antibiotics, and pesticide residues, and dairy becomes a major driver of systemic inflammation.

6. Peanuts - Highly susceptible to aflatoxin contamination, a potent liver toxin and carcinogen [13]. Their high lectin content damages the gut lining, while their 30-40% oil content contributes to omega-6 overload and inflammatory cascades.

7. Industrial seed oils - Canola, soybean, corn, sunflower, safflower, and cottonseed oils now comprise 20% of American calories, up from zero a century ago [14]. These oils are high in omega-6 fatty acids, prone to oxidation, and create toxic aldehydes when heated, causing mitochondrial dysfunction and inflammation.

8. Alcohol - A Group 1 carcinogen according to the WHO, with no safe level of consumption [15]. Alcohol damages the gut lining, overwhelms liver detoxification, disrupts sleep architecture, and impairs mitochondrial function. The social

acceptance of alcohol obscures its role as a major driver of chronic disease.

9. Chemical additives and preservatives - The average American consumes 140-150 pounds of additives per year, up from 2 pounds in 1900. These include emulsifiers that destroy gut bacteria, preservatives that disrupt hormones, artificial colors linked to behavioral problems, and flavor enhancers that override satiety signals.

Why This Book Is Different

You might be thinking, 'Another diet book? Haven't we been down this road before?' And you'd be right to be skeptical. The diet industry generates $72 billion annually selling temporary solutions to permanent problems [16]. But this isn't a diet book in the traditional sense. This is a restoration manual for your body's operating system.

First, this approach is based on understanding mechanisms, not following rules. When you understand why certain foods trigger MILA dysfunction leading to chronic illness, the choices become obvious. You are not avoiding foods because someone told you they're 'bad'; you're eliminating specific substances that demonstrably interfere with cellular function. This is not about moral judgments or food fear; it's about biological compatibility.

Second, this is a systematic protocol, not random restrictions. The order matters. The preparation matters. The implementation matters. Too many people fail not because the approach is wrong, but because they try to do everything at once or skip critical steps. This book provides a roadmap that ensures success by working with your body's healing sequence, not against it.

Third, this addresses root causes, not symptoms. While medications might temporarily suppress symptoms, they often worsen the underlying dysfunction. Proton pump inhibitors for acid reflux increase intestinal permeability [17]. Statins for cholesterol deplete CoQ10, crucial for mitochondrial function [18]. NSAIDs for pain damage the gut lining and impair healing [19]. We need a different approach, one that restores function rather than suppressing dysfunction.

Finally, this book bridges the gap between complex science and practical application. You will understand the biology, but more importantly, you'll know exactly what to do about it. From meal planning to restaurant navigation, from handling social situations to managing cravings, this book provides the practical tools that make implementation possible in the real world.

Maria's Transformation: What's Possible When You Restore the Terrain

Remember Maria from the beginning of this chapter? Her transformation illustrates what is possible when you address root causes rather than chase symptoms. We started by eliminating the

Toxic Nine, but not all at once. First went the sugar and processed foods, then the gluten and dairy, finally the seed oils and hidden additives. Each phase brought improvements, but the real magic happened when all nine categories were removed.

Within two weeks, her brain fog began lifting. 'It was like someone cleaned my windshield,' she told me. 'I didn't realize how cloudy everything had become until it cleared.' By week four, her joint pain had decreased by 70%. She could open jars again, write on the board without wincing, and play with her students during recess. Her digestive issues, which had plagued her for fifteen years, completely resolved within six weeks.

But the transformation went beyond symptom relief. Her energy returned, not the jittery, caffeine-fueled energy she'd been surviving on, but deep, sustained energy that lasted all day. Her mood stabilized. Her sleep deepened. She lost 23 pounds without counting calories or feeling hungry. Most remarkably, lab tests that had been 'borderline' for years normalized. Her inflammatory markers dropped to optimal levels. Her thyroid function improved. Her hormone balance restored.

The gastroenterologist who had dismissed her concerns as 'just IBS' was stunned. The rheumatologist who had been preparing to start her on immune-suppressing biologics told her to keep doing whatever she was doing. Even her family doctor, initially skeptical of the dietary approach, asked for information to share with other patients. Maria did not just get her health back; she got her life back.

Eighteen months later, Maria remains symptom-free. She's not perfect with the protocol, she'll have a piece of birthday cake at special celebrations or enjoy a meal out without interrogating the waiter. But she understands her body now, knows what triggers problems, and has the tools to quickly restore balance when needed. She has become an advocate in her school, quietly revolutionizing the lunch program and teaching her students about real food. 'I spent fifteen years looking for answers in medicine,' she says, 'when the answer was on my plate all along.'

How to Use This Book

This book is structured to take you on a journey from understanding to implementation. The early chapters establish the scientific foundation, explaining what has happened to our food supply and why it matters for your health. You'll learn about each of the Toxic Nine in detail, understanding not just what to avoid but why these foods trigger such profound dysfunction. This is not about memorizing lists; it is about developing intuition for what serves your biology and what sabotages it.

The middle chapters transition from theory to practice. You will learn how to navigate the real world, from grocery shopping to eating out, from handling social pressure to managing cravings. We'll address the psychological aspects of dietary change, because knowing what to eat is only half the battle; the other half is doing it consistently in a world designed to make you fail.

The later chapters address common challenges and special circumstances. What about food sensitivities beyond the Toxic Nine? How do you handle holidays and special occasions? What if you're an athlete with higher energy needs? What about children, pregnancy, or elderly parents? We will cover it all, ensuring you have the tools to adapt the protocol to your unique situation.

Throughout, you'll find patient stories that illustrate key concepts. These aren't just success stories meant to inspire; they are teaching cases that show how the protocol applies to different conditions, challenges, and life circumstances. You will see yourself in these stories and understand that you are not alone in this journey. This is not just a book; it's a complete system for transformation.

To properly progress through the protocol, you will want more personalized guidance. The Dynamic Intake assessment at restoremila.com can help identify your specific patterns and priorities, providing customized recommendations based on your unique biology and circumstances. While this book provides the foundation, the assessment offers fine-tuning that optimizes your results.

Understanding how we got here is crucial for recognizing why change is necessary. The transformation of our food supply did not happen overnight; it was a gradual process that accelerated dramatically in recent decades.

In the next chapter, we will explore this transformation in detail, seeing how foods that sustained humanity for millennia became the very substances now destroying our health. What you'll discover is both shocking and enlightening, revealing that our current health crisis isn't a mystery but a predictable consequence of treating food as an industrial commodity rather than biological necessity.

Key Takeaways:

Modern chronic disease is not a mystery; it's the predictable result of eating foods our bodies do not recognize as food.

The MILA protocol, encompassing mitochondrial, immune, and lymphatic function, determines whether we maintain health or develop disease.

The R.E.S.T.O.R.E. MILA protocol provides a systematic approach to healing that works with biology rather than against it.

The Toxic Nine categories of inflammatory foods must be eliminated for the body to restore normal function.

This isn't another diet; it's a restoration protocol that addresses root causes rather than suppressing symptoms.

Chapter 1:

The Great Food Transformation - How We Got Here

Robert walked into my office carrying two grocery bags to show me what he was eating. They were filled with what he considered 'healthy' foods. At 58, a recently retired engineer who had spent his career solving complex problems, he could not understand why he couldn't solve his own health crisis. Type 2 diabetes, high blood pressure, sixty pounds of excess weight, and chronic fatigue had crept up on him over two decades. 'I eat better than I did in college,' he said, unpacking whole grain bread, low-fat yogurt, granola bars, and diet soda. 'I choose the healthy options. I read labels. I avoid fast food. So why do I keep getting worse?'

Robert's confusion was entirely justified. He was doing everything the food pyramid, his doctor, and conventional wisdom had told him to do. He'd switched from white bread to whole wheat, from regular soda to diet, from butter to margarine and then to 'heart-healthy' vegetable oils. He counted calories, chose low-fat options, and exercised when his energy allowed. Yet his hemoglobin A1c kept climbing, his inflammation markers stayed elevated, and he needed more medications each year to manage conditions that seemed to multiply like weeds in an untended garden.

What Robert did not understand, and what most people don't understand, is that the foods he considered healthy bore little resemblance to the foods our grandparents ate, despite carrying the same names. The 'whole wheat' bread contained dwarf wheat hybridized for yield, not nutrition, with gluten levels that would have been impossible in traditional varieties. The yogurt was made from milk produced by cows that were fed genetically modified corn and soy, treated with hormones and antibiotics, then processed until it barely resembled dairy. The granola bars contained more sugar than a candy bar, just hidden under names like brown rice syrup, agave nectar, and evaporated cane juice. Even the vegetables in his refrigerator had been bred for shelf life and appearance, not nutritional content, and were coated with waxes and preservatives he couldn't pronounce.

The Speed of Change: When Evolution Met Revolution

To understand our current health crisis, we need to grasp the unprecedented speed at which our food supply has changed. Human beings have been on Earth for approximately 300,000 years. For 299,900 years, we ate foods that came directly from nature: animals we hunted, fish we caught, plants we gathered, and eventually, crops we grew. The foods changed with seasons and locations, but their fundamental nature remained constant. They were whole, unprocessed, and recognizable.

The industrial revolution began changing this around 150 years ago, but the real transformation has occurred in just the last 50-70 years. To put this in perspective, if human existence were compressed into a single year, the industrial food system would have emerged in the last second of that year. In evolutionary terms, we have given our bodies less than a second to adapt to completely foreign substances. Is it any wonder they are rebelling?

Consider wheat, a grain humans have cultivated for 10,000 years. Traditional wheat varieties like einkorn and emmer stood four to five feet tall, contained 14 chromosomes, and had gluten contents around 2-4% [20]. Through natural selection and basic farming practices, these grains sustained civilizations from ancient Egypt to medieval Europe. Then, in the 1960s, everything changed.

The Green Revolution, led by Norman Borlaug, introduced dwarf wheat varieties that revolutionized agriculture. These new strains, created through intensive chemical mutagenesis and crossbreeding, stood only two feet tall, contained 42 chromosomes, and had gluten contents exceeding 12% [21]. They could produce twice the yield per acre, resist lodging (falling over), and respond dramatically to synthetic fertilizers. Borlaug won the Nobel Peace Prize for preventing famine, and his varieties now comprise 95% of wheat grown worldwide [22].

But this agricultural triumph came with unintended consequences. The new wheat contained novel proteins never before encountered by human digestive systems. The gliadin proteins were restructured in ways that increased their ability to trigger zonulin release, the protein that regulates intestinal permeability [23]. Where traditional wheat fermentation through sourdough broke down problematic proteins and anti-nutrients, modern industrial bread-making uses fast-acting yeast and chemical dough conditioners, leaving these inflammatory compounds intact [24].

The Sugar Revolution: From Rare Treat to Metabolic Poison

Perhaps no food has undergone a more dramatic transformation than sugar. In 1700, the average person consumed approximately 4 pounds of sugar per year, and that was only if they were wealthy enough to afford it [25]. Sugar was a luxury item, sold in locked boxes in apothecaries, prescribed medicinally in small doses. It was so valuable that it was called 'white gold,' and wars were fought over sugar-producing territories.

Fast forward to today: the average American consumes 152-170 pounds of sugar annually, a 3,000-4,000% increase [8]. This isn't just from obvious sources like candy and soda. Sugar hides under 61 different names in 74% of packaged foods [26]. It's in your pasta sauce (often more sugar than ice cream topping), your 'healthy' smoothie (up to 60 grams per serving), your salad dressing, your bread, even your deli meat. Food manufacturers have weaponized our evolutionary preference for sweetness, originally designed to identify ripe, nutritious fruits, and turned it into a tool for creating addiction and driving consumption.

Patricia, a 45-year-old accountant, discovered this hidden sugar trap when she started reading labels carefully. 'I was shocked,' she told me. 'My breakfast of whole grain cereal with skim milk and orange juice contained 67 grams of sugar. That is more than 16 teaspoons before 8 AM. My 'light' yogurt had more sugar than a Snickers bar. My protein bar that I thought was healthy contained corn syrup, brown rice syrup, and cane sugar, simply different names for the same poison.' When we calculated her daily intake, she was consuming over 180 grams of sugar daily while believing she ate healthfully.

The explosion in sugar consumption directly parallels the rise in metabolic disease. In 1890, the death rate from diabetes was 2.8 per 100,000 people. By 2020, it had increased to over 25 per 100,000, and that's just deaths, not diagnoses [27]. Type 2 diabetes, once so rare in children it was called 'adult-onset diabetes' now affects millions of young people. Non-alcoholic fatty liver disease, unknown before 1980, now affects 25-30% of Americans [28].

But sugar's damage extends beyond simple caloric excess. When consumed in current quantities, sugar triggers a cascade of metabolic dysfunction. It glycates proteins, creating Advanced Glycation End products (AGEs) that damage tissues throughout the body [29]. It feeds pathogenic bacteria and yeasts in the gut, disrupting the microbiome [30]. It suppresses white blood cell function for hours after consumption, weakening immune defenses [31]. It triggers dopamine release in the brain's reward centers, creating addiction patterns similar to cocaine [32].

The Rise of GMOs: Rewriting the Code of Life

In 1994, the Flavr Savr tomato became the first genetically modified organism (GMO) approved for human consumption. Marketed as a tomato that would stay fresh longer, it seemed like a benign innovation. But it opened the floodgates to a transformation of our food supply that makes the Green Revolution look conservative by comparison. Within two decades, GMOs would dominate American agriculture.

Today, 92% of corn, 94% of soybeans, and 96% of cotton (whose oil ends up in food) grown in the United States is genetically modified [11]. These are not crops that have been selectively bred over generations; they've had genes from completely different species inserted into their DNA. Corn has been engineered to produce its own pesticide, containing genes from Bacillus thuringiensis (Bt) that cause insects' stomachs to explode [33]. Soybeans have been modified to survive being drenched in herbicides that would kill natural plants.

The biotech industry assured us these modifications were safe, that the Bt toxin would be destroyed in human digestion, that glyphosate (the herbicide most GMOs are designed to resist) was harmless to humans. But research tells a different story. The

Bt toxin has been found in the blood of 93% of pregnant women and 80% of their unborn babies [34]. Glyphosate, originally patented as an antibiotic, disrupts the gut microbiome and has been linked to cancer, leading to billions in lawsuit settlements [35].

William, a 67-year-old retired military officer, experienced firsthand how GMOs can affect health. 'I grew up on a farm,' he said. 'We raised our own corn, wheat, and vegetables. I could eat anything without problems. Then I spent thirty years eating military and processed food. By the time I retired, I had developed severe digestive issues, joint pain, and chronic sinusitis. My doctor said it was just aging.' When we eliminated GMO foods from his diet, his symptoms began resolving within weeks. 'It wasn't aging,' he realized. 'It was the food.'

The GMO issue isn't about the genetic modifications themselves. These crops enable and encourage massive herbicide use. Glyphosate application has increased 15-fold since GMO crops were introduced [36]. This chemical doesn't just stay on the fields; it persists in the food supply. Testing has found glyphosate residues in everything from breakfast cereals to wine, from infant formula to honey [37]. We are conducting an uncontrolled experiment on the human population, and the early results are alarming.

The Seed Oil Revolution: From Machine Lubricant to 'Heart-Healthy' Food

One of the most dramatic yet overlooked transformations in our food supply has been the replacement of traditional fats with industrial seed oils. For all human history, we consumed fats from animals (butter, tallow, lard) and fruits (olive oil, coconut oil, avocado oil). These fats were minimally processed, stable at cooking temperatures, and compatible with human biology. Then, in the early 1900s, everything changed.

The story begins with Procter & Gamble, a soap and candle company looking for a cheaper alternative to animal fats. In 1907, they discovered that cotton seed oil, a toxic waste product of the cotton industry, could be chemically altered through hydrogenation to create a solid fat that resembled lard. They called it Crisco, marketed it as 'a healthier alternative to animal fats,' and gave away free cookbooks to promote its use [38]. It was the beginning of a revolution that would fundamentally alter the American diet.

The real push came in the 1960s when Ancel Keys' flawed Seven Countries Study seemed to link saturated fat to heart disease [39]. Despite cherry-picked data and ignored contradictions, his hypothesis became dogma. The American Heart Association, influenced by funding from Procter & Gamble and other oil manufacturers, began recommending polyunsaturated vegetable oils over traditional fats [40]. Suddenly, butter was poison and margarine was medicine.

Today, soybean oil alone accounts for 7% of American calories [41]. When you add in corn oil, canola oil, sunflower oil, and other industrial seed oils, they comprise approximately 20% of the American diet, up from essentially zero in 1900 [42]. These oils are in everything: salad dressings, mayonnaise, baked goods, restaurant food, even products labeled as 'healthy' or 'organic.' They are so ubiquitous that avoiding them requires careful label reading and often means avoiding most prepared foods.

The processing required to create these oils should give us pause. Seeds are heated to extreme temperatures, pressed with tremendous force, extracted with hexane (a petroleum derivative), de-gummed with phosphoric acid, neutralized with sodium hydroxide, bleached with chlorine, and deodorized at temperatures exceeding 400°F [43]. The resulting product is so far removed from food that it requires artificial colors and flavors to make it palatable. Compare this to traditional olive oil production: crush olives, collect oil. Which sounds more like food?

These oils fundamentally alter our biology. They're extremely high in omega-6 fatty acids, creating an inflammatory imbalance in the body. Our ancestors consumed omega-6 to omega-3 ratios around 2:1 or 3:1. Today's ratio often exceeds 20:1, driving systemic inflammation [44]. When heated, these oils produce toxic aldehydes and lipid peroxides that damage cellular membranes, particularly in mitochondria [45]. They're literally oxidizing us from the inside out.

The Chemical Invasion: 7,000% More Additives

In 1900, Americans consumed approximately two pounds of chemical food additives per year, mostly basic preservatives like salt and natural compounds like vinegar [46]. Today, that number has exploded to 140-150 pounds annually, a 7,000% increase [47]. The FDA's Generally Recognized as Safe (GRAS) list contains over 10,000 approved additives, most of which have never been tested for long-term human consumption [48].

These are not just preservatives to prevent spoilage. They are emulsifiers that allow oil and water to mix in processed foods but destroy the protective mucus layer in our intestines [49]. They are artificial colors derived from petroleum that have been linked to hyperactivity in children [50]. They're flavor enhancers that override our natural satiety signals, causing us to overeat [51]. They are texture modifiers, stabilizers, anti-caking agents, and dozens of other categories of chemicals that have turned food into a chemistry experiment.

Consider a simple comparison: your grandmother's bread contained flour, water, yeast, and salt. Today's commercial bread can contain over 30 ingredients, including calcium propionate (linked to autism-like behaviors in children), azodicarbonamide (also used in yoga mats and shoe rubber), potassium bromate (banned in Europe and Canada as a carcinogen), and high fructose corn syrup (because apparently bread needs added sugar) [52].

The cumulative effect of these chemicals is impossible to study because no one consumes just one additive. We are exposed to hundreds daily, creating infinite possible interactions. What we do know is alarming. Emulsifiers like polysorbate-80 and carboxymethylcellulose, common in ice cream and baked goods, have been shown to promote inflammatory bowel disease and metabolic syndrome [53]. Artificial sweeteners, marketed as healthy alternatives to sugar, disrupt gut bacteria and may promote diabetes [54].

The Nutrient Decline: More Food, Less Nutrition

While we have been adding chemicals to our food, we've simultaneously been stripping away nutrients. This isn't just about processing; even whole foods have experienced dramatic nutrient declines. A landmark study comparing nutrient data from 1950 to 1999 found significant decreases in protein, calcium, phosphorus, iron, riboflavin, and vitamin C in 43 different vegetables and fruits [55].

Modern agricultural practices prioritize yield, shelf life, and appearance over nutrition. Tomatoes are picked green and artificially ripened with ethylene gas, preventing the development of lycopene and other nutrients [56]. Apples are bred for sweetness and crunch, not vitamin content. Some modern sweet corn varieties contain 40% sugar, compared to 3% in heritage varieties [57]. We are eating more food but getting less nutrition, a recipe for simultaneous obesity and malnutrition.

Soil depletion compounds the problem. Intensive farming has stripped soils of minerals, and synthetic fertilizers only replace nitrogen, phosphorus, and potassium, not the dozens of trace minerals plants need to produce nutrients [58]. A carrot grown in depleted soil might look like a carrot, but it lacks the magnesium, zinc, and other minerals that made carrots nutritious in the first place.

The Blue Zones: Living Proof of What We've Lost

While Americans experience skyrocketing rates of chronic disease, five regions of the world, known as Blue Zones, maintain remarkable health and longevity. In Okinawa, Japan; Sardinia, Italy; Nicoya, Costa Rica; Ikaria, Greece; and Loma Linda, California, people routinely live to 100 with minimal chronic disease [59]. What is their secret? They eat food that has not been transformed by modern industrial processing.

In these regions, people still consume traditional foods prepared in traditional ways. Their wheat is often ancient varieties, fermented or sprouted before consumption. Their dairy, when consumed, comes from grass-fed animals and is often fermented. They eat minimal sugar, no industrial seed oils, and virtually no processed foods. They don't count calories or follow fad diets; they simply eat real food.

The contrast is striking. In Ikaria, where people eat wild greens, herbal teas, raw honey, and traditionally prepared grains, the rate of dementia is 75% lower than in the United States [60].

In Okinawa, eating sweet potatoes, seaweed, and small amounts of traditionally raised pork, the rate of heart disease is 80% lower [61]. These are not genetic anomalies; when people from Blue Zones adopt Western diets, they develop Western diseases at Western rates [62].

Robert's Awakening: Seeing Through the Marketing

As Robert learned about the transformation of our food supply, his engineer's mind began connecting dots. 'I've been debugging complex systems my entire career,' he said. 'But I never thought of debugging my diet. I assumed food was food, that an apple was an apple, that bread was bread. I trusted the labels, the marketing, the authorities telling me what was healthy.

We went through his bags of groceries together, reading labels with new understanding. His 'whole grain' cereal contained 37 ingredients, including three types of sugar and BHT, a petroleum derivative also used in embalming fluid. His 'heart-healthy' margarine was a cocktail of inflammatory seed oils, emulsifiers, and artificial flavors. His low-fat salad dressing compensated for the missing fat with high fructose corn syrup and chemical thickeners. Even his vitamin supplements contained artificial colors, titanium dioxide, and other questionable additives.

'This isn't food,' Robert said quietly, surveying his purchases. 'This is a chemistry experiment. No wonder my body is breaking down. I'm not giving it anything it recognizes as nourishment.' The revelation was both disturbing and liberating. Disturbing because he realized how badly he had been deceived. Liberating because now he knew what to do about it.

Robert's transformation began with a simple principle: eating foods your great-grandmother would recognize. Out went the processed foods, the industrial oils, the hidden sugars. In came whole foods: grass-fed meats, wild-caught fish, organic vegetables, nuts, seeds, and fruits. The change was not easy, but it was profound. Within three months, his blood sugar normalized. His blood pressure dropped. He lost 31 pounds without counting calories. Most remarkably, his energy returned. 'I feel like I'm aging in reverse,' he said six months later. 'All from eating real food.'

The Perfect Storm: When All Changes Converged

Each transformation we've discussed would be challenging enough for human biology to adapt to individually. But they did not happen in isolation. They converged over the same 50–70-year period, creating a perfect storm of dietary disruption. We simultaneously increased sugar consumption by 3,000%, replaced traditional fats with industrial oils, genetically modified our staple crops, and added thousands of chemicals to our food supply. We stripped nutrients while adding toxins. We turned food from nourishment into poison.

The human body is remarkably resilient. It can handle occasional insults, temporary nutritional deficiencies, and short-term toxic exposures. But it cannot handle constant, multiple, simultaneous attacks on its fundamental operating systems. When every meal contains inflammatory oils, excessive sugar, modified proteins, and chemical additives, the body never gets a chance to recover. The damage accumulates, systems begin failing, and chronic disease becomes inevitable.

This explains why we are seeing diseases in children that used to only affect the elderly. It explains why multiple chronic conditions are becoming the norm rather than the exception. It explains why healthcare costs are spiraling out of control despite medical advances. We are not dealing with mysterious new diseases; we're dealing with the predictable consequences of feeding human bodies substances they were never designed to process.

Now that we understand how dramatically our food has been transformed, we need to examine the specific categories of foods causing the most damage. The Toxic Nine represents the worst offenders in our modern food supply, each triggering specific mechanisms of dysfunction in the MILA system. In the next chapter, we will dive deep into the first three: sugar, wheat, and corn, understanding exactly how these seemingly innocent foods have been weaponized against our biology. What you will learn will forever change how you look at that morning toast, afternoon snack, or evening dessert.

Key Takeaways:

Our food supply has undergone a radical transformation in just 50-70 years, a timeframe that represents less than 0.03% of human evolution.

Sugar consumption has increased 3,000%, wheat has been hybridized beyond recognition, over 90% of corn and soy is genetically modified, industrial seed oils have replaced traditional fats, and chemical additives have increased 7,000%.

These changes happened simultaneously, creating a perfect storm of metabolic disruption.

Blue Zones demonstrate that traditional diets still produce remarkable health and longevity.

The solution is not complicated: return to eating real, whole foods that our bodies recognize as nourishment.

Chapter 2:

The Toxic Nine

Part 1: Sugar, Wheat, and Corn

Anthony walked into my office holding his head in his hands, something he had been doing a lot lately. At 34, this brilliant software developer who had built two successful companies could not think straight anymore. 'It's like my brain is wrapped in cotton,' he told me. 'I'll see how to fix a problem, then two seconds later, it's gone. I'll write code and immediately forget why I wrote it. I've tried everything — special brain supplements, tons of coffee, meditation, exercise. Nothing helps.

His problems had started small five years ago — just feeling tired in the afternoons, which he blamed on working too much. But it kept getting worse until he could barely function. He had seen twelve different doctors. The brain specialist found nothing wrong with his MRI. The psychiatrist said he was burned out and gave him antidepressants. The hormone doctor said his levels were 'normal.' The functional medicine doctor had him taking forty-seven different supplements that cost a fortune and made him feel sick but did not clear his head. He'd spent over $30,000 trying to fix himself, yet no one had really looked at what he was eating every day.

When we went through his food diary together, I immediately saw the problem, though he couldn't. His 'healthy' morning smoothie had 67 grams of sugar from fruit, honey, and protein powder - that is like eating 17 sugar cubes for breakfast. His whole wheat sandwich at lunch sent his blood sugar soaring, then crashing. His afternoon 'energy' bar was basically a candy bar pretending to be healthy. He was on a sugar roller coaster all day long, and it was destroying his brain. But it was worse than just sugar — these three foods were attacking his body's basic operating system, what I call the MILA system. The sugar was shutting down his energy production, the wheat was breaking down his gut barrier, and the corn was poisoning his cells with GMO proteins and pesticides.

Sugar: The Sweet Poison Hiding Under 61 Different Names

Sugar is especially dangerous because it attacks all three parts of your MILA system at once. Let me explain what MILA means in simple terms. Your mitochondria are like tiny power plants in every cell that make energy. Your immune system is like your body's army, protecting you from invaders. Your lymphatic system is like your body's garbage disposal and drainage system. When these three systems work together properly, you feel great. When sugar damages them, everything starts breaking down.

At the cellular level, sugar basically caramelizes your proteins - imagine what happens when you heat sugar in a pan until it turns brown and sticky. That's happening inside your body, creating damaged proteins called AGEs [29]. Your immune system sees these damaged proteins as invaders and stays on high alert, creating inflammation. Meanwhile, your lymphatic system gets clogged trying to clean up all this cellular garbage, leading to swelling, brain fog, and exhaustion.

The food industry knows sugar is addictive and harmful, so they hide it using 61 different names. Most people have no idea how they're eating sugar when they see these names on labels [63].

Here is the complete list everyone needs to know:

Agave nectar	Barley malt and barley malt syrup
Beet sugar	Brown rice syrup
Brown sugar	Cane juice, cane juice crystals, and cane sugar
Caramel	Carob syrup
Coconut sugar and coconut palm sugar	Corn sweetener and corn syrup
Date sugar	Dextrin and dextrose
Evaporated cane juice	Fructose
Fruit juice and fruit juice concentrate	Galactose
Glucose	Golden syrup

High fructose corn syrup	Honey
Invert sugar	Lactose
Malt syrup	Maltodextrin
Maltose	Maple syrup
Molasses and blackstrap molasses	Muscovado
Palm sugar	Panela and panocha
Raw sugar and organic raw sugar	Rice syrup and rice bran syrup
Saccharose	Sorghum syrup
Sucrose	Treacle
Turbinado sugar	

And many more variations like buttered syrup, castor sugar, confectioner's sugar, crystalline fructose, demerara sugar, Florida crystals, grape sugar, icing sugar, mannose, powdered sugar, rapadura, refiner's syrup, sucanat, sweet sorghum, tapioca syrup, yellow sugar, and xylose.

Food companies use a sneaky trick called 'ingredient splitting.' They will use four or five different types of sugar in one product. That way, sugar doesn't appear as the first ingredient, even if you added them all up, sugar would be the main ingredient. Your 'healthy' granola bar might list oats first, but then have honey, brown rice syrup, cane juice, and maple syrup scattered throughout the ingredient list. You are eating mostly sugar without knowing it.

When you eat sugar, your body releases insulin to deal with it. But here is what most people don't know: when insulin stays high all the time from eating sugar constantly, it actually stops your cells from making new mitochondria — those energy power plants I mentioned [64]. Without enough mitochondria, your cells cannot make energy properly. They are forced to use a backup system that only produces two units of energy instead of the normal 36 units. No wonder you feel exhausted!

This energy crisis hits your brain especially hard. Even though your brain is only 2% of your body weight, it uses 20% of your energy. When your mitochondria cannot keep up, your brain starts shutting down non-essential functions. First, you lose creativity. Then complex thinking gets hard. Finally, you can't even form new memories properly. This is exactly what happened to Anthony - not from aging or stress, but from sugar destroying his cellular power plants.

Sugar also wrecks your immune system. Studies show that eating 75 grams of sugar — about two cans of soda - cuts your white blood cell function in half for five hours [65]. These are the cells that fight infections and cancer. If you are eating sugar at every meal and snack, your immune system never fully recovers. You're basically turning off your body's defense system several times a day.

The lymphatic system damage is just as bad. Sugar feeds bad bacteria and yeast in your gut, especially Candida, which produces toxins your lymph system has to clean up [66]. At the same time, sugar makes your lymph fluid thick and sticky by increasing fat levels in your blood. It's like trying to drain a sink with honey instead of water — everything backs up. This creates the puffiness, brain fog, and constant feeling of being 'toxic' that so many people experience.

Denise, a 41-year-old marketing executive, discovered this sugar-MILA connection the hard way. 'I was exhausted all the time, even sleeping nine hours a night,' she told me. 'I'd have a vanilla latte and blueberry muffin for breakfast, crash by 10 AM, grab another coffee and a protein bar — which was really just a candy bar with protein added. By 3 PM, I needed chocolate just to stay awake.' When we tested her, she was producing less than half the cellular energy she should have been. Her immune system was constantly activated, and her lymph nodes were swollen and congested. She was literally drowning in sugar-created waste while her cells starved for energy.

Why Sugar Substitutes Make Things Worse, Not Better

When people learn how bad sugar is, their first thought is usually: 'I'll just use artificial sweeteners instead!' But here's the problem — these substitutes can actually be worse than sugar for your MILA system. Let me explain why, and what these substitutes actually are.

Common artificial sweeteners include aspartame (Equal, NutraSweet), sucralose (Splenda), saccharin (Sweet'N Low), acesulfame potassium (Ace-K, Sunett), neotame, and advantame.

'Natural' alternatives include stevia, monk fruit, erythritol, xylitol, sorbitol, mannitol, and allulose. While these sound healthier because they are 'natural,' they still cause major problems in your body.

Here's what happens: when your tongue tastes something sweet - ANY sweet taste - it sends a signal to your brain saying, 'Sugar is coming!' Your brain then tells your pancreas to release insulin to deal with the expected sugar [54]. Your stomach makes more acid. Your liver gets ready to process glucose. Your cells prepare to receive fuel. But with artificial sweeteners, no actual sugar arrives. Your body is all dressed up with nowhere to go.

This creates chaos in your MILA system. Your mitochondria are waiting for fuel that never comes, wasting energy staying in 'ready mode.' Unnecessary insulin makes your blood sugar drop, causing intense cravings for real sugar. Your immune system sees this confusion as a danger signal and stays activated. Your lymphatic system has to clean up all the hormones that were released for no reason. You end up more inflamed and tired than if you had just eaten regular sugar.

Artificial sweeteners also destroy your gut bacteria even worse than sugar does. Studies show they can kill up to half your good bacteria in just a few weeks [67]. These good bacteria are crucial for making vitamins, supporting your immune system, and even producing brain chemicals that affect your mood. When they die off, bad bacteria take over, producing toxins that inflame your gut and overwhelm your lymph system.

Some artificial sweeteners break down into poisons in your body. Aspartame turns into formaldehyde - yes, embalming fluid - and methanol, which is wood alcohol [68]. These toxins accumulate in your brain, heart, and liver, damaging your mitochondria's DNA. Even 'natural' sugar alcohols like xylitol can ferment in your gut, feeding bad bacteria and causing bloating, gas, and diarrhea.

The solution is not to find a 'safe' sugar substitute - it is to retrain your taste buds completely. Here is the amazing part: your taste buds replace themselves every 10-14 days. When you stop eating anything sweet - including artificial sweeteners - for just 30 days, something magical happens. Your taste buds reset to their natural sensitivity. Suddenly, carrots taste sweet. Almonds have a delightful sweetness. Even lettuce has a subtle sweet flavor you never noticed. This is how your body is supposed to work before food companies hijack your taste buds for profit.

Modern Wheat: The Mutant Grain That Even Bugs Won't Eat

Growing up in the 1970s, I have vivid memories of my grandmother's kitchen rituals. She kept her flour in heavy metal canisters with tight-fitting lids, and before baking, she'd always sift it carefully through a fine mesh screen. 'What are you looking for, Grandma?' I once asked. 'Weevils,' she said matter-of-factly, picking out the tiny beetles that always seemed to find their way into the flour. 'Bugs love real food. If bugs won't eat something, neither should you.'

Fast forward to today. I can leave a bag of modern flour open on my kitchen counter for months - even years - and not a single bug will touch it. The flour looks the same, smells the same, has the same name on the package. But it's been so fundamentally changed that even insects - who will eat almost anything organic - recognize it as non-food. When bugs will not eat something, that's nature's warning label. This transformation of wheat has devastating effects on your MILA system.

Modern wheat attacks your body through multiple pathways. The main troublemaker is a protein called gliadin, which triggers your gut to release something called zonulin [69]. Think of zonulin as the key that opens the doors between your intestinal cells. Normally, these doors stay tightly closed, only letting in fully digested nutrients. But when wheat triggers zonulin, the doors fly open, allowing partially digested food, bacteria, and toxins to flood into your bloodstream. Your immune system goes crazy trying to fight all these invaders, your lymph system gets overwhelmed trying to clean up the mess, and your mitochondria get damaged by all the inflammation.

The wheat our great-grandparents ate was completely different from what we eat today. Ancient wheat had 14 chromosomes (think of these as instruction manuals for the plant) and was tall, reaching 4-5 feet high. It had about 2-4% gluten. In the 1960s, scientists used chemicals and radiation to create a mutant dwarf wheat with 42 chromosomes [22]. This new wheat is only 2 feet tall and contains 12-14% gluten that is 3 to 6 times more than traditional wheat! This wasn't slow, natural change over thousands of years. This was creating a Frankenstein grain in a laboratory.

But here is something that makes modern wheat even more toxic that most doctors don't know we produce much less stomach acid than our ancestors did. By age 40, we make 30% less acid, and by 60, we are down by half [70]. Why? Chronic stress shuts down acid production. Antacids and acid blockers, which millions take daily, reduce it further. Common nutrient deficiencies, especially zinc and B vitamins, impair our ability to make acid. And half the population has H. pylori bacteria, which damages the cells that produce stomach acid.

Without enough stomach acid, wheat proteins don't get broken down properly. Instead of being digested into individual amino acids that your body can use, they remain as larger chunks that your body sees as foreign invaders. These partially digested wheat proteins act like morphine in your brain [71]. They are called gluteomorphins, and they bind to the same receptors as heroin and morphine. This is why people get genuine withdrawal symptoms when they stop eating wheat - anxiety, depression, brain fog, and intense cravings. It is also why food companies put wheat in everything; they know it's addictive.

Modern wheat also contains something called wheat germ agglutinin, or WGA, which is the plant's natural insecticide [72]. WGA is incredibly tough — it survives cooking, stomach acid, and digestive enzymes completely intact. Once it gets into your bloodstream, it sticks to your cells like glue, especially in your joints (causing arthritis-like pain), your thyroid (disrupting hormones), and your mitochondria. When WGA attaches to mitochondria, it punches holes in their membranes, causing them to leak. It's like poking holes in a battery — the energy just drains out.

Traditional cultures knew wheat needed special preparation. They fermented their bread dough for days using wild yeast (sourdough), which broke down the gluten, neutralized the WGA, and pre-digested the grain [24]. Modern bread is made in under 3 hours using commercial yeast and dozens of chemicals. None of the toxic proteins get broken down. We are eating wheat in the most toxic form possible.

George, a 55-year-old contractor, discovered wheat's devastating effects firsthand. 'I developed rheumatoid arthritis at 45, just like my dad and grandfather,' he told me. 'Within five years, I couldn't grip my tools. My hands were so swollen I couldn't make a fist. The drugs my rheumatologist gave me suppressed my immune system so badly that I caught every cold that went around.' When we tested him, his zonulin levels were three times normal - his gut was wide open. His cellular energy production was down 60%. His lymph system was completely congested, especially around his inflamed joints. Three weeks after eliminating wheat, his morning stiffness went from three hours to thirty minutes. After three months, his pain was down 70% and his energy had returned.

Corn: The GMO Trojan Horse That's Poisoning Your Energy System

If sugar floods your system and wheat breaks down your barriers, corn delivers the final blow by directly poisoning your mitochondria. Remember, mitochondria are your cellular power plants. The GMO proteins in corn act like tiny bombs that blow holes in these power plants, causing them to leak and fail [33]. This is not science fiction — it is happening in your body every time you eat corn products.

Today, 92% of corn grown in America is genetically modified [73]. The most common type is called Bt corn, which has genes from bacteria inserted into it. Every single cell of this corn produces its own pesticide — a poison designed to kill insects by destroying their stomachs. The biotech companies promised this was safe because they said the poison would be destroyed by human stomach acid. They lied.

Scientists have found these Bt toxins in the blood of 93% of pregnant women and 80% of their unborn babies [34]. This proves the toxins survive digestion and even cross into the womb. Once in your blood, these bacterial proteins attack your mitochondria using the same mechanism they use to kill insects — they punch holes in cell membranes. Imagine your mitochondria as tiny batteries, and these proteins are like drill bits making holes in them. The batteries leak can't hold a charge and eventually die [74].

Here's exactly how Bt proteins damage your mitochondria: they target a special fat molecule called cardiolipin that is only found in mitochondrial membranes [75]. Cardiolipin is like the scaffolding that holds the energy-production machinery in place. When Bt proteins destroy cardiolipin, the whole energy production system falls apart. Your cells try to compensate by using backup energy systems, but these only produce 2 units of energy instead of 36. This is why people eating GMO corn feel constantly exhausted — their cellular batteries are literally leaking.

High fructose corn syrup (HFCS) attacks your MILA system differently. Unlike regular sugar, which every cell in your body can use, fructose can only be processed by your liver. When you drink a soda with 50-75 grams of HFCS, it is like dumping a truckload of toxic waste on your liver [76]. Your liver's mitochondria get overwhelmed and start producing dangerous free radicals - think of them as cellular rust. The liver turns excess fructose into fat, leading to fatty liver disease, which now affects 30% of Americans. A fatty liver can't detoxify your body properly, so toxins build up everywhere.

Corn oil makes things even worse. It contains omega-6 fats in a ratio of 46 to 1 compared to omega-3s [77]. Your ancestors ate these fats in a 2 to 1 ratio. This massive imbalance creates inflammation throughout your body. These inflammatory fats get built into your cell membranes, making them stiff and dysfunctional. When corn oil is heated for cooking, it produces toxic chemicals that specifically destroy the first step in your mitochondria's energy production line [78]. It's like removing the first gear from an engine — nothing else can work properly.

GMO corn is also soaked in glyphosate (Roundup), which does not wash off because it's absorbed into every cell of the plant [79]. Glyphosate works like a molecular thief, stealing essential minerals your mitochondria need to function. It grabs onto manganese, magnesium, iron, and zinc — all critical for energy production. Without these minerals, your mitochondria can't complete their energy cycles. It also kills your good gut bacteria, which produce vitamins and other compounds your mitochondria need. You are being poisoned from multiple directions at once.

Corn hides in thousands of products under names you'd never recognize. Citric acid, vitamin C, xanthan gum, maltodextrin, dextrose, MSG — all typically derived from corn. Even if you think you're avoiding corn, you're probably eating it multiple times every day, keeping your mitochondria under constant attack.

The Triple Threat: How Sugar, Wheat, and Corn Work Together to Destroy Your Health

While each of these foods is harmful alone, together they create a perfect storm of destruction in your body. Think of it like this: sugar is flooding your house, wheat is breaking down the walls, and corn is setting everything on fire. Your body's systems cannot handle this triple attack.

Here's what happens when you eat a typical breakfast cereal. Within minutes, wheat triggers zonulin, opening your gut barrier like opening floodgates. Now corn's Bt toxins and partially digested proteins rush into your bloodstream. Your immune system freaks out, releasing inflammatory chemicals that damage your mitochondria even more. Meanwhile, sugar shuts down half of your white blood cells right when you need them most. Your lymph system tries to clean up this disaster but gets overwhelmed and backs up like a clogged drain. Each food makes the others more toxic, creating damage that takes days to recover from — but recovery never comes because lunch and dinner deliver the same combination.

The lack of stomach acid makes everything worse. Those partially digested wheat and corn proteins are like sending half-built, sharp-edged Lego blocks through your system instead of smooth, finished pieces. They cause maximum damage and inflammation. Sugar suppresses your immune system so it cannot properly deal with these foreign proteins. The corn oil amplifies all the inflammation. It's like throwing gasoline on a fire while trying to put it out with a garden hose that's been turned down to a trickle.

Anthony's Amazing Recovery: Proof Your Body Can Heal

When Anthony eliminated sugar, wheat, and corn from his diet, his body began healing immediately. 'The first week was absolute hell,' he admitted. 'Splitting headaches, intense cravings, felt like I had the flu. But this was actually my body finally being able to clean out years of toxic buildup. My lymph system was like a dam breaking - finally able to drain. By day ten, I woke up and it was like someone had cleaned a dirty window I'd been looking through for years. The brain fog was completely gone.'

Lab tests confirmed what he was feeling. His cellular energy production increased by 65% in just six weeks. His zonulin levels normalized, showing his gut barrier had healed. Inflammatory markers that had been sky-high for years dropped to normal. Lymphatic imaging showed clear drainage for the first time. 'I realized I hadn't lost my intelligence,' he said. 'I'd been poisoning my brain three times a day, every day, for years. My body knew how to heal - I just had to stop poisoning it.'

Six months later, Anthony wasn't just back to normal, he was better than ever. His energy lasted from morning to night without any crashes. His coding productivity didn't just return; it tripled. The anxiety and depression he had battled for years completely disappeared. 'I spent $30,000 on fancy supplements and medications trying to fix my brain. The real solution did not cost anything. I just had to stop eating three foods that were destroying my cellular power plants, inflaming my immune system, and clogging my drainage system.'

Sugar, wheat, and corn are just the first three of the Toxic Nine foods destroying your health. While removing these three can dramatically improve your energy and clear your brain, complete healing requires eliminating all nine. In the next chapter, we'll expose three more troublemakers: soy, dairy, and peanuts.

You'll discover why that 'healthy' soy protein is scrambling your hormones worse than any drug, why dairy products are triggering autoimmune attacks throughout your body, and why peanuts contain natural toxins so dangerous that even cancer researchers use them to cause liver tumors in lab studies.

Key Takeaways:

Sugar hides under 61 different names and attacks your energy system, immune function, and lymphatic drainage all at once.

Modern wheat is a mutant grain that even bugs won't eat, triggering leaky guts and acting like morphine in your brain, made worse by our reduced stomach acid.

GMO corn produces bacterial toxins that punch holes in your cellular batteries while drowning your liver in fructose.

Sugar substitutes trick your body into chaos without providing any benefit.

These three foods work together, each making the others more toxic, creating a perfect storm of cellular destruction that explains why so many people feel exhausted, inflamed, and sick.

Chapter 3:

The Toxic Nine

Part 2: Soy, Dairy, and Peanuts

Helen walked into my office with a thick folder documenting her five-year battle with Hashimoto's thyroiditis. At 48, a yoga instructor who taught six classes a week and followed what she believed was an exemplary plant-based diet, she couldn't understand why her body was attacking its own thyroid. 'I've eliminated meat, I drink soy milk, eat tofu daily, and have protein shakes made with soy protein isolate,' she explained. 'I'm doing everything right according to every health magazine, but my antibodies keep climbing and my symptoms keep worsening.

Her dedication to 'healthy' eating was admirable but misguided. Her daily soy latte delivered 25 grams of soy protein isolate. Her lunch typically included tofu or tempeh. Her snacks were soy-based protein bars. She consumed 60-80 grams of soy protein daily, believing she was protecting her health. In reality, she was flooding her system with phytoestrogens, enzyme inhibitors, and one of the most genetically modified, pesticide-laden crops in America.

Beyond the soy, her 'clean' diet included Greek yogurt for probiotics, string cheese for calcium, and peanut butter for healthy fats and protein. Each of these foods, marketed as nutritious, was contributing to her autoimmune cascade through different mechanisms. Her story illustrates a critical truth: foods that seem healthy according to conventional wisdom can be driving the very diseases we're trying to prevent.

What Helen did not understand was how these foods were systematically dismantling her MILA system. Her mitochondria were trapped in Cell Danger Response, unable to produce adequate energy. Her immune system was chronically activated, creating antibodies against her own thyroid tissue. Her lymphatic system was congested, unable to clear the inflammatory debris that accumulated daily. Each soy shake, each bowl of yogurt, each spoonful of peanut butter added fuel to this dysfunctional fire.

Soy: The Hormone Disruptor Masquerading as Health Food

Soy has achieved a reputation as a health food based on observations of traditional Asian diets, where soy consumption is associated with lower rates of certain cancers and heart disease. But there's a critical distinction that's been lost in translation: traditional Asian cultures consume primarily fermented soy in small quantities, while Americans consume unfermented, highly processed soy in amounts that would astonish anyone from Japan or China.

In Asia, soy consumption averages 10-20 grams per day, mostly as fermented products like miso, natto, and tempeh [80]. The fermentation process neutralizes anti-nutrients, breaks down problematic proteins, and creates beneficial compounds. These foods are consumed as condiments, not as primary protein sources. Contrast this with American consumption: a single soy protein shake can contain 25-40 grams of unfermented soy protein isolate, and many health-conscious Americans consume multiple soy products daily.

The problems begin with how soy is grown. In the United States, 94% of soy is genetically modified to withstand heavy applications of glyphosate [81]. This means nearly all non-organic soy products contain residues of this herbicide, now linked to cancer, microbiome disruption, and mineral chelation that creates functional deficiencies [82]. Think of glyphosate as a battering ram against your MILA system. It damages mitochondrial membranes, disrupts the gut bacteria that regulate your immune system, and binds to minerals your cells need to function.

Your mitochondria struggle to produce energy, your immune system becomes confused, and your lymphatic system can't clear the toxic load.

Even organic soy is not exempt from problems; it still contains the natural anti-nutrients and hormone disruptors inherent to the bean. Soy contains the highest levels of phytoestrogens of any food, particularly isoflavones like genistein and daidzein [83]. These compounds mimic estrogen in the body, binding to estrogen receptors and triggering estrogenic effects. While marketed as beneficial for menopausal symptoms, the reality is more complex and concerning.

Here's what happens to your MILA system when phytoestrogens flood your body: Your mitochondria, which have estrogen receptors on their membranes, receive confusing signals that disrupt normal energy production. Your immune system becomes dysregulated because sex hormones directly influence immune cell function, creating the conditions for autoimmune disease. Your lymphatic vessels, which also respond to hormonal signals, become sluggish and congested. The result is a cascade of dysfunction that conventional medicine calls 'hormonal imbalance' but is actually MILA collapse disguised as endocrine issues.

For women, excessive soy consumption can disrupt menstrual cycles, worsen PMS, contribute to infertility, and potentially promote estrogen-dependent cancers [84]. For men, studies have shown that high soy intake can reduce testosterone levels, decrease sperm count, and even cause gynecomastia (male breast development) [85]. For children, soy formula delivers the estrogenic equivalent of 3-5 birth control pills daily, potentially affecting sexual development and future fertility [86].

Victor, a 39-year-old fitness trainer, learned about soy's hormonal effects the hard way. 'I switched to plant-based protein powders, mainly soy, thinking it was healthier than whey,' he said. 'Within six months, my testosterone dropped from 680 to 340 ng/dL. I lost muscle mass, gained belly fat, had zero libido, and developed mild gynecomastia. My doctor wanted to put me on testosterone replacement. Instead, I eliminated soy and my levels recovered to 625 within four months.'

Victor's recovery wasn't just about testosterone. When we tested his cellular function, we found something remarkable: his mitochondrial ATP production increased by 40% after eliminating soy. His inflammatory markers normalized. His lymphatic congestion resolved. The hormone disruption was just the visible symptom of deeper MILA dysfunction.

Soy also contains potent enzyme inhibitors, particularly trypsin inhibitors, which interfere with protein digestion [87]. These inhibitors can survive cooking and processing, arriving intact in your digestive system where they block the enzymes needed to break down proteins. This leads to protein malabsorption, digestive distress, and increased allergic potential as undigested proteins trigger immune responses. When your body can't properly digest protein, your immune system sees these large, undigested protein fragments as foreign invaders, triggering inflammation and antibody production. This is MILA dysfunction at the gut level, where immune activation begins.

The goitrogenic compounds in soy present another problem, particularly for thyroid health. These compounds interfere with iodine uptake by the thyroid gland, potentially leading to hypothyroidism and goiter [88]. For someone like

Helen with existing thyroid issues, consuming large amounts of soy was like throwing gasoline on a fire. The very food she thought was helping was exacerbating her autoimmune thyroid condition.

The thyroid is incredibly energy-intensive, requiring optimal mitochondrial function to produce hormones. When soy compounds block iodine, your thyroid cells must work harder to capture what little iodine is available. This increased metabolic demand pushes already stressed mitochondria deeper into Cell Danger Response. The immune system, sensing this cellular stress, increases its surveillance of the thyroid tissue, eventually creating the antibodies that define Hashimoto's thyroiditis.

Understanding this mechanism reveals why conventional thyroid treatment often fails. Doctors prescribe thyroid hormone replacement, which provides temporary symptomatic relief but doesn't address the underlying MILA dysfunction. The mitochondria in thyroid cells remain stressed. The immune attack continues. The goitrogenic compounds from soy keep blocking iodine uptake. The patient feels marginally better but never truly heals, requiring increasing medication doses over time as their thyroid tissue is progressively destroyed. This is management, not healing. True healing requires removing the triggers that initiated MILA collapse in the first place.

Perhaps most concerning is how soy is processed into the products Americans consume. Soy protein isolate, found in protein powders, bars, and meat substitutes, is created through a highly industrial process involving hexane extraction, acid washing, and high-temperature processing [89]. This creates denatured proteins, removes beneficial compounds, concentrates anti-nutrients, and can form toxic lysinoalanine and nitrosamines. You're not eating a bean; you're eating an industrial product that happens to originate from a bean. These processing chemicals themselves damage mitochondria, trigger immune reactions, and add to your body's toxic burden that must be cleared through an already overwhelmed lymphatic system.

Dairy: The Inflammatory Cascade Hidden in Every Glass

Dairy holds a sacred place in American nutrition mythology. The milk mustache campaigns, the food pyramid's dairy requirements, the insistence that children need milk for strong bones; all of this has created an unquestioned belief that dairy is essential for health. But for 65-70% of the global population who are lactose intolerant, and the millions more who react to dairy proteins, this 'essential' food is actually a major driver of inflammation and disease [90].

The problems with modern dairy begin with the cows themselves. Through selective breeding, we've created Holstein cows that produce 10 times more milk than their ancestors [91]. These cows predominantly produce A1 beta-casein, a protein that didn't exist in original cattle breeds. When A1 beta-casein is digested, it produces beta-casomorphin-7 (BCM-7), an opioid peptide that can cross the intestinal barrier and even the blood-brain barrier [92].

BCM-7 acts like morphine in the body, binding to opioid receptors and triggering a cascade of effects: inflammation, immune dysregulation, altered gut motility, and even behavioral changes [83]. This is why dairy can be literally addictive, why children have meltdowns when dairy is removed, and why adults experience withdrawal symptoms. It's also why dairy is linked to conditions ranging from Type 1 diabetes to autism to heart disease [94].

From a MILA perspective, BCM-7 is a perfect storm of dysfunction. This opioid peptide binds to receptors on immune cells, altering their response patterns and creating the chronic immune activation that depletes energy and overwhelms the lymphatic system. It crosses into the brain, affecting mitochondrial function in neurons and disrupting the signals that regulate inflammation. It slows gut motility, allowing bacterial overgrowth that produces toxins requiring lymphatic clearance. One glass of milk initiates a cascade that reverberates through your entire MILA system for hours.

Natalie, a 52-year-old nurse, discovered dairy's inflammatory effects after years of unexplained symptoms. 'I had chronic sinus infections, joint pain, acne at 52, and digestive issues I'd accept as normal,' she told me. 'I drank milk for calcium, ate yogurt for probiotics, and had cheese daily. When I eliminated dairy, it was like someone turned off an inflammation switch. sinuses cleared in a week, joints stopped aching in two weeks, skin cleared completely in a month. Twenty years of antibiotics for sinus infections, and the solution was to stop drinking milk.

Natalie's rapid improvement reveals an important truth about MILA restoration: when you remove a major inflammatory trigger, the system can rebalance surprisingly quickly. Her lymphatic congestion resolved, allowing accumulated inflammatory debris to clear. Her immune system downregulated, reducing antibody production against her own tissues. Her mitochondria emerged from Cell Danger Response, resuming normal energy production. The chronic sinus infections weren't caused by bacteria; they were caused by dairy-induced immune dysfunction creating an environment where bacteria could thrive.

What's fascinating about Natalie's case is how interconnected her symptoms were, though they seemed unrelated on the surface. Sinus infections, joint pain, acne, and digestive issues appear to involve completely different body systems. But through the MILA lens, they're all manifestations of the same root dysfunction. The dairy proteins triggered immune activation. The chronic immune activation depleted mitochondrial energy. The reduced energy impaired lymphatic flow. The sluggish lymphatic system couldn't clear inflammatory mediators from her sinuses, joints, or skin. Everything was connected through MILA, and removing dairy allowed the entire system to restore balance simultaneously. This is why people often report improvement in seemingly unrelated symptoms when they eliminate major food triggers; they're not treating separate conditions, they're restoring integrated system function.

Lactose intolerance, affecting the majority of adults worldwide, is actually the normal state. The ability to digest lactose into adulthood is a recent genetic mutation that occurred in some populations about 7,500 years ago [95]. For the billions who lack this mutation, consuming dairy means flooding the colon with undigested lactose, feeding pathogenic bacteria, creating gas, bloating, diarrhea, and systemic inflammation from bacterial endotoxins. These endotoxins are precisely what trigger mitochondrial Cell Danger Response, creating the fatigue and brain fog that people accept as 'normal aging' but is actually dairy-induced MILA dysfunction.

Modern processing makes dairy even more problematic. Pasteurization, while preventing acute infections, denatures proteins, destroys enzymes that aid digestion, and kills beneficial bacteria [86]. Homogenization breaks fat globules into microscopic particles that can bypass normal digestion and enter the bloodstream directly, carrying proteins and hormones deep into tissues where they trigger immune responses [96]. Your immune system wasn't designed to encounter milk proteins in your bloodstream; when it does, it appropriately treats them as foreign invaders, creating inflammation and antibodies.

The hormone content of modern dairy is another concern. Dairy cows are kept pregnant nearly continuously to maintain milk production, resulting in milk with high levels of estrogen and progesterone [97]. They're also treated with recombinant bovine growth hormone (rBGH) to increase production, leading to elevated IGF-1 levels in milk. IGF-1

(Insulin-like Growth Factor 1) promotes cell proliferation and is linked to increased cancer risk, particularly breast, prostate, and colorectal cancers [88].

These hormones don't just affect reproductive tissues. They directly impact your MILA system. IGF-1 pushes cells toward growth and proliferation, requiring massive amounts of ATP. When your mitochondria are already struggling, this increased energy demand deepens their dysfunction. Cancer cells essentially hijack this growth signal while simultaneously switching to glycolytic metabolism that produces more inflammatory byproducts. The lymphatic system, already overwhelmed, cannot clear the increased cellular debris from rapid cell turnover.

The pesticide and antibiotic residues in conventional dairy add another layer of toxicity. Cows concentrate toxins in their milk, acting as bioaccumulators of whatever chemicals are in their feed and environment. Testing has found pesticides, antibiotics, heavy metals, and even flame retardants in milk samples [89]. These compounds disrupt hormones, damage mitochondria, and contribute to antibiotic resistance. Each glass of conventional milk delivers a cocktail of chemicals that your liver must detoxify, your lymphatic system must clear, and your mitochondria must defend against.

Even organic, grass-fed dairy isn't exempt from problems. While it may have better fatty acid profiles and fewer toxins, it still contains casein proteins, lactose, and natural hormones that many people cannot tolerate. The idea that switching to 'better' dairy solves the problem is like switching from regular cigarettes to organic ones; you are still consuming something inherently problematic for many people.

Peanuts: The Toxic Legume Masquerading as a Nut

Peanuts occupy a unique position in the American diet. They're in everything from candy bars to cooking oils, from school lunches to bar snacks. Americans consume over 6 pounds of peanuts per person annually, mostly as peanut butter [90]. But peanuts aren't actually nuts; they are legumes that grow underground, and this distinction matters tremendously for your health.

Growing underground makes peanuts uniquely susceptible to contamination with Aspergillus mold, which produces aflatoxins, among the most carcinogenic substances known to science [91]. Aflatoxins are so toxic that they're classified as Group 1 carcinogens by the International Agency for Research on Cancer, the same category as asbestos and plutonium [92]. While the FDA sets 'acceptable' levels for aflatoxin in peanuts, the reality is that there is no safe level of a carcinogen.

Studies have found that 37-45% of peanut samples contain detectable aflatoxins, with some exceeding safety limits [93]. These toxins accumulate in the body over time, particularly in the liver where they can cause cellular mutations leading to hepatocellular carcinoma. They also suppress immune function, interfere with nutrient absorption, and contribute to growth stunting in children. Countries with high peanut consumption have correspondingly high rates of liver cancer.

Aflatoxins are mitochondrial poisons. They directly damage the electron transport chain, the cellular machinery that produces ATP. When your mitochondria encounter aflatoxins, they immediately enter Cell Danger Response, shutting down normal metabolism to prevent further damage. Your immune system recognizes these damaged, stressed cells and increases surveillance, creating inflammation. Your liver, working overtime to detoxify aflatoxins, produces inflammatory byproducts that must be cleared through your lymphatic system. That 'healthy' peanut butter sandwich is a MILA disruptor disguised as protein.

Beyond aflatoxins, peanuts contain exceptionally high levels of lectins, proteins that plants use as a defense mechanism against predators [94]. Peanut lectin is particularly resistant to digestion and cooking, surviving the journey through your digestive system intact. Once in the gut, these lectins bind to the intestinal lining, damaging the protective mucus layer and increasing intestinal permeability. They can also enter circulation and bind to tissues throughout the body, triggering autoimmune responses.

This is leaky gut in action. When peanut lectins damage your intestinal barrier, larger food particles, bacteria, and toxins can cross into your bloodstream. Your immune system, encountering these molecules where they shouldn't be, creates antibodies and inflammation. This systemic immune activation keeps your MILA system in a perpetual state of alert, unable to restore normal function.

Many people do not realize they have intestinal permeability until they develop obvious autoimmune symptoms. But the damage begins long before diagnosis. Every time you eat peanut butter on toast, those lectins are quietly eroding your gut barrier. The immune cells stationed along your intestinal wall detect the breach and sound the alarm. Your mitochondria, responding to immune signals, reduce energy production and increase defensive measures. Your lymphatic vessels in the gut wall, called lacteals, become inflamed and congested. Over months and years, this daily assault creates the chronic MILA dysfunction that eventually manifests as recognizable disease. The peanut butter sandwich seems innocent, but it's a slow-motion catastrophe for sensitive individuals.

The omega-6 content of peanuts presents another problem. Peanuts are approximately 30-40% oil by weight, predominantly omega-6 fatty acids with no omega-3s [98]. This contributes to the inflammatory imbalance that characterizes the modern diet. When you consume peanut butter daily, you're adding fuel to the inflammatory fire that drives chronic disease. Omega-6 fatty acids are converted into inflammatory signaling molecules called prostaglandins and leukotrienes, which tell your immune system to remain activated and prevent your lymphatic system from resolving inflammation.

Peanuts are also one of the most common food allergens, affecting approximately 1-2% of the population with reactions ranging from mild itching to life-threatening anaphylaxis [99]. But beyond true allergies, many more people have peanut sensitivities that manifest as digestive issues, skin problems, joint pain, or respiratory symptoms. The proteins in peanuts are particularly allergenic, with Ara h 1, 2, and 3 being major allergens that can trigger severe reactions even in minute quantities.

The processing of peanuts into peanut butter often makes them even more problematic. Commercial peanut butter contains added sugars, inflammatory seed oils, and emulsifiers to prevent separation. Even 'natural' peanut butter is often made from peanuts roasted at high temperatures, which increases aflatoxin formation and creates acrylamide, another carcinogen [96]. The convenience of peanut butter has made it a dietary staple, but it's a staple that's slowly poisoning many people.

The agricultural practices used in peanut farming compound these issues. Peanuts are one of the most pesticide-intensive crops, with residues of multiple chemicals found in tested samples [97]. These pesticides don't just sit on the surface; because peanuts have soft, porous shells, chemicals penetrate the legume itself. Washing or choosing organic helps but doesn't eliminate the inherent problems with peanuts.

Helen's Transformation: Reversing Autoimmunity by Eliminating the Hidden Triggers

When Helen eliminated soy, dairy, and peanuts from her diet, along with the sugar, wheat, and corn we'd previously addressed, her transformation was remarkable. 'The first thing I noticed was my energy,' she said. 'Within two weeks, I didn't need my afternoon nap. The brain fog I'd attributed to thyroid dysfunction lifted. But the real shock came at my three-month follow-up.

Her thyroid antibodies, which had been climbing steadily for five years despite medication, dropped by 60%. Her TSH normalized without increasing her thyroid medication. Her inflammatory markers fell into optimal range. The joint pain she'd accepted as part of aging disappeared. Most surprisingly to her, the anxiety and mood swings she'd battled since her thirties completely resolved.

What happened inside Helen's body during those three months reveals the power of MILA restoration. Without the constant assault of soy phytoestrogens, dairy proteins, and peanut lectins, her mitochondria emerged from Cell Danger Response. ATP production increased, providing the energy her immune cells needed to function properly rather than chaotically. Her immune system, no longer constantly triggered by food antigens, down-regulated its attack on her thyroid tissue. Her lymphatic system, freed from the burden of clearing inflammatory debris from reactive foods, could finally clear the backlog of toxins and cellular waste that had accumulated over years.

'I'd been a vegetarian for ethical reasons,' Helen reflected, 'but I was relying so heavily on soy and dairy that I was destroying my health. I've added back clean animal proteins, and for the first time in years, I feel genuinely healthy. My yoga practice has transformed; I have flexibility and strength I haven't had since my thirties. My students keep asking what I'm doing differently.

Six months after eliminating these foods, Helen's Hashimoto's was in complete remission. Her antibodies were undetectable, her thyroid function had normalized, and she was able to reduce her medication by half. Her endocrinologist, initially skeptical of the dietary approach, now refers patients to learn about the protocol. 'He told me he's never seen antibodies drop like mine did,' Helen said. 'He asked for copies of everything I was doing to share with other patients.'

Helen's story illustrates a fundamental truth about MILA-based healing: when you remove what's blocking the system and give it time to restore function, the body's innate healing capacity is extraordinary. Her thyroid wasn't permanently broken; it was under siege. Her immune system wasn't defective; it was responding appropriately to the constant inflammatory signals from foods she consumed daily. Her fatigue wasn't inevitable aging; it was mitochondrial shutdown from chronic stress.

Soy, dairy, and peanuts complete the protein portion of the Toxic Nine, but three more categories remain that are equally destructive to the MILA system. In the next chapter, we'll explore the final trio: seed oils that oxidize your cells from within, alcohol that's toxic at any dose, and the thousands of chemical additives that have turned our food into a chemistry experiment.

These last three are the most insidious because they hide in foods we don't suspect and accumulate damage slowly over years. Understanding how they dismantle your MILA system will complete your ability to identify and eliminate the foods that stand between you and optimal health.

Key Takeaways:

Soy, dairy, and peanuts create MILA dysfunction through multiple mechanisms.

Soy floods the system with phytoestrogens that disrupt mitochondrial signaling, enzyme inhibitors that trigger immune reactions, and glyphosate residues that damage cellular function.

Dairy delivers opioid peptides that dysregulate immune responses, inflammatory proteins that keep the system on high alert, and hormones that push mitochondria beyond their capacity.

Peanuts harbor aflatoxins that poison mitochondrial energy production, lectins that breach the intestinal barrier triggering systemic immune activation, and inflammatory omega-6 oils that prevent resolution of inflammation.

These three foods are particularly deceptive because they're marketed as healthy protein sources while systematically dismantling the MILA system.

When eliminated, many people experience dramatic improvements in energy, immunity, and inflammatory conditions within weeks as their mitochondria emerge from Cell Danger

Response, their immune systems rebalance, and their lymphatic systems clear accumulated debris.

The speed of recovery reveals that the body isn't broken; it's simply overwhelmed by foods that trigger constant MILA dysfunction.

Chapter 4

The Toxic Nine

Part 3: Seed Oils, Alcohol, and Chemical Additives

Richard's Invisible Poison

Richard walked into my office looking like someone had beaten him from the inside out. At 44 years old, this successful restaurant owner had built a thriving farm-to-table establishment that won awards for its commitment to fresh, locally sourced ingredients. He was the last person who should have been sick. Yet he sat, 35 pounds heavier than he'd been five years ago, with fatty liver disease, chronic joint inflammation, and a persistent brain fog that made managing his business increasingly difficult. 'I don't understand,' he said, frustration evident in his voice. 'I eat better than anyone I know. We source everything from local farms. I haven't eaten fast food in twenty years.

Richard's confusion was understandable. By conventional standards, he was doing everything right. His restaurant served grass-fed beef, free-range chicken, and organic vegetables. He avoided processed foods. He didn't drink sodas or eat candy. Yet his labs told a disturbing story: liver enzymes elevated three times normal, inflammatory markers through the roof, triglycerides dangerously high, and markers of oxidative stress that suggested his mitochondria were under constant assault.

The answer to Richard's mystery lay not in what foods he was eating, but in how those foods were being prepared. His kitchen, like every restaurant kitchen in America, relied on industrial seed oils for cooking. Vegetable oil for high heat. Canola oil for dressings. Soybean oil in marinades. His staff went through gallons of these oils daily, and Richard himself consumed them with every meal he ate at his own restaurant. He was also a 'moderate' drinker, enjoying two or three glasses of wine with dinner most evenings, a habit his doctor had encouraged as 'heart healthy.' And despite his commitment to fresh ingredients, the reality of restaurant operations meant his food still contained countless chemical additives, from the 'natural flavors' in his spice blends to the emulsifiers in his dairy products.

Richard was unknowingly poisoning himself with the final three members of the Toxic Nine, the very substances that complete the picture of modern dietary destruction. While sugar, wheat, corn, soy, dairy, and peanuts do immense damage, these last three, seed oils, alcohol, and chemical additives, may be the most insidious of all because they hide in everything we consume.

Seed Oils, The Fat That Changed Everything

If you want to understand how dramatically human health has declined in the past century, you need to look no further than the transformation of our fat consumption. In 1900, the average American consumed virtually zero industrial seed oils. These products simply did not exist. Our ancestors cooked with butter, lard, tallow, and occasionally olive oil — fats that humans had consumed for thousands of years. Today, seed oils constitute approximately 20 percent of all calories consumed by Americans, representing the single largest change to the human diet in evolutionary history [42].

The story of how this happened reveals everything that's wrong with modern nutrition science and food manufacturing. In the early 1900s, Procter & Gamble developed a process called partial hydrogenation that could transform liquid cottonseed oil, previously used primarily for lamp fuel and industrial applications, into a solid fat that resembled lard [100]. The company marketed this industrial product as Crisco, positioning it as a modern, scientific alternative to traditional animal fats. It was cheaper to produce, had an indefinite shelf life, and could be manufactured in unlimited quantities. The fact that human beings had never consumed it before was presented as an advantage rather than a warning.

The American Heart Association's fateful decision in the 1960s to recommend vegetable oils over saturated fats, based largely on flawed research funded by the sugar industry, opened the floodgates [40]. Suddenly, these industrial products were not just acceptable but actively recommended. Food manufacturers rushed to replace traditional fats with cheaper seed oils. Restaurants discovered they could save money by switching from expensive animal fats to inexpensive vegetable oils. Within a generation, seed oils went from zero percent of the American diet to the dominant source of fat calories.

The industrial seed oils that now dominate our food supply, including soybean oil, canola oil, corn oil, sunflower oil, safflower oil, cottonseed oil, and grapeseed oil, share several characteristics that make them uniquely destructive to human health. They are all extracted through industrial processes involving high heat, chemical solvents like hexane, and extensive refining that strips away any protective compounds while concentrating problematic ones [40]. They are all extremely high in omega-6 polyunsaturated fatty acids, particularly linoleic acid. And they are all highly susceptible to oxidation, meaning they become toxic when exposed to heat, light, or oxygen.

The Omega-6 Catastrophe

The human body requires both omega-6 and omega-3 fatty acids, but the ratio matters enormously. Throughout human evolution, our ancestors consumed these fats in roughly equal proportions, with ratios ranging from 1:1 to perhaps 4:1 omega-6 to omega-3 [44]. This balance allowed the body to use omega-6 fatty acids for their intended purpose, producing inflammatory signals when needed for wound healing and infection fighting, while omega-3 fatty acids provided the anti-inflammatory signals to resolve inflammation once the threat had passed. The system worked beautifully for millions of years.

Today, the average American consumes omega-6 and omega-3 fatty acids in a ratio of approximately 15:1 to 20:1 [101]. Some individuals, particularly those who eat out frequently or consume large amounts of processed foods, have ratios exceeding 25:1. This represents a fundamental distortion of human biochemistry, a shift so extreme that our cellular machinery simply cannot compensate.

When omega-6 fatty acids dominate the diet to this degree, the consequences are predictable and devastating. The body produces inflammatory signaling molecules called eicosanoids in excess while being unable to produce adequate anti-inflammatory compounds [98]. Chronic inflammation becomes the default state rather than an occasional response to injury or infection. Every tissue in the body suffers: joints become inflamed, blood vessels develop atherosclerosis, brain tissue accumulates inflammatory damage, and the immune system becomes perpetually activated.

The mitochondrial damage from excess omega-6 consumption is particularly severe. These polyunsaturated fats incorporate into mitochondrial membranes, where they are highly vulnerable to oxidative damage [102]. When these membrane fats oxidize, they produce toxic aldehydes that damage mitochondrial DNA and impair energy production. Research has shown that elevated linoleic acid consumption directly correlates with markers of mitochondrial dysfunction and cellular energy deficiency [103]. The very organelles that should be powering your cells become damaged by the fats in your diet.

Aldehydes: The Toxic Byproducts

The destruction wrought by seed oils extends far beyond omega-6 imbalance. When these highly unstable fats are heated, as they are in virtually every cooking application, they undergo rapid oxidation and produce a class of compounds called aldehydes [104]. These molecules, including 4-hydroxynonenal (4-HNE) and malondialdehyde (MDA), are among the most toxic substances you can consume.

Research has demonstrated that the aldehyde content of seed oils heated to typical cooking temperatures exceeds the concentrations found in cigarette smoke [105].

4-HNE deserves particular attention because it has been identified as a primary driver of multiple degenerative diseases. This compound forms covalent bonds with proteins, DNA, and cellular membranes, essentially creating molecular damage that accumulates over time [102]. Studies have linked 4-HNE to Alzheimer's disease, Parkinson's disease, atherosclerosis, liver disease, and cancer [106]. Every time you consume food cooked in seed oils, you ingest these compounds and accelerate the aging and degeneration of your tissues.

The restaurant industry presents a particular problem in this regard. Commercial deep fryers maintain seed oils at high temperatures for extended periods, often reusing the same oil for days. With each heating cycle, the aldehyde content increases dramatically [107]. Studies of commercial frying oils have found aldehyde concentrations hundreds of times higher than in fresh oil. When Richard ate meals at his own restaurant, even though the ingredients were high quality, he was consuming these toxic compounds with every bite of anything that had been fried or roasted in his kitchen's vegetable oils.

The Liver Burden

Richard's fatty liver disease was no coincidence. The liver bears the primary burden of processing dietary fats, and the explosion of seed oil consumption has overwhelmed this organ in ways never before seen in human history. Non-alcoholic fatty liver disease (NAFLD), virtually unknown before 1980, now affects approximately 25 percent of the global population [28]. Among Americans, the prevalence exceeds 30 percent and continues to climb.

The connection between seed oils and fatty liver disease is now well established. Linoleic acid, the primary omega-6 fat in seed oils, is preferentially stored in the liver where it promotes fat accumulation and inflammatory damage [108]. Animal studies have demonstrated that diets high in soybean oil produce more severe fatty liver disease than diets high in saturated fat, even when total fat content and calories are identical [109]. The type of fat matters more than the amount, and seed oils are the worst possible choice for liver health.

The progression from fatty liver to non-alcoholic steatohepatitis (NASH) to cirrhosis to liver cancer has become one of the most common pathways to serious illness in the developed world [110]. What makes this particularly tragic is that it is entirely preventable. Simple elimination of seed oils and replacement with traditional fats like olive oil, coconut oil, butter, and animal fats can reverse early-stage fatty liver disease within months.

Angela's Transformation

Angela was 36 years old, a marketing manager who prided herself on eating 'healthy.' She cooked at home using 'heart-healthy' canola oil, packed salads with dressings made from soybean oil, and avoided butter and animal fats religiously. She could not understand why she kept gaining weight despite eating only 1,400 calories per day, or why her inflammatory markers kept climbing despite her 'anti-inflammatory' diet. 'I've done everything the nutritionists tell me to do,' she said. 'I've eliminated red meat, I use vegetable oils instead of butter, I eat whole grains. Why am I getting sicker?

Angela's story illustrates how thoroughly bad science has corrupted nutritional guidance. She had followed the official recommendations perfectly, and those recommendations were making her ill. When we analyzed her diet, we found she consumed approximately 40 grams of linoleic acid daily, nearly all of it from seed oils [111]. Her omega-6 to omega-3 ratio was

22:1. Her liver ultrasound showed moderate fatty infiltration despite the fact that she rarely drank alcohol.

We eliminated all seed oils from Angela's diet and replaced them with olive oil for dressings, coconut oil, and butter for cooking, and encouraged her to eat fatty fish twice weekly. We actually increased her total fat intake while dramatically shifting the composition. Within three months, Angela had lost 18 pounds without reducing her caloric intake. Her inflammatory markers dropped by 60 percent. Her fatty liver began to resolve. She was eating more fat than ever before, but she was eating the right fats.

Alcohol, The Terrain Destroyer

Richard's nightly wine habit represented what his previous doctors had actually encouraged, a 'moderate' drinking pattern supposedly associated with longevity and heart health. The so-called 'French Paradox,' the observation that French people had lower rates of heart disease despite consuming saturated fat, was attributed to their wine consumption. For decades, medical professionals have told patients that moderate alcohol consumption is not only safe but actively beneficial. This advice is wrong, and the scientific evidence now conclusively demonstrates that no level of alcohol consumption is safe for health [112].

The supposed benefits of moderate drinking have been thoroughly debunked by careful analysis of the original studies. The apparent health advantage of moderate drinkers over abstainers largely disappeared when researchers controlled for a critical confounding factor: many 'abstainers' were former heavy drinkers who had quit due to health problems [113]. When only lifetime abstainers were compared to moderate drinkers, the health advantage vanished. Additionally, moderate drinkers tend to be wealthier, better educated, and have better access to healthcare than abstainers, all factors that independently predict better health outcomes.

The World Health Organization's International Agency for Research on Cancer has classified alcohol as a Group 1 carcinogen, the same category as asbestos, tobacco smoke, and plutonium [114]. This is not a preliminary finding or a controversial opinion. It represents the scientific consensus based on overwhelming evidence. Alcohol causes at least seven types of cancer: mouth, throat, esophagus, liver, colon, rectum, and breast [115]. The risk begins at any level of consumption and increases with dose. There is no safe threshold.

Acetaldehyde: The Real Poison

When you consume alcohol, your liver converts it first to acetaldehyde and then to acetate. While acetate is relatively harmless, acetaldehyde is one of the most toxic compounds your body will ever encounter. It is approximately 30 times more toxic than alcohol itself [116]. This compound damages DNA, impairs cellular repair mechanisms, disrupts mitochondrial function, and creates widespread oxidative stress. The damage it causes is cumulative and often irreversible.

The liver can only process acetaldehyde at a limited rate, meaning that the more alcohol you consume, the longer this toxic compound circulates in your system [117]. Even 'moderate' consumption of two glasses of wine produces acetaldehyde levels that persist for hours after drinking ends. During this time, the compound is actively damaging tissues throughout your body. The familiar symptoms of a hangover are actually symptoms of acetaldehyde poisoning.

For Richard, his years of 'moderate' drinking had produced measurable damage. His liver, already stressed by seed oil consumption, showed signs of alcoholic inflammation superimposed on his fatty liver disease [118]. His gut permeability testing revealed significant intestinal barrier dysfunction. His inflammatory markers told the story of chronic, low-grade poisoning from a substance his doctors had told him was healthy.

Alcohol and the MILA System

The destruction alcohol wreaks on the Mitochondrial-Immune-Lymphatic Axis is systematic and severe. Each component of MILA suffers direct damage, and the combined effect creates a cascade of dysfunction that accelerates aging and promotes chronic disease.

Mitochondria are particularly vulnerable to alcohol and its metabolites. Acetaldehyde directly damages mitochondrial DNA, which lacks the protective histones and repair mechanisms that protect nuclear DNA [119]. Studies have demonstrated that even moderate alcohol consumption reduces mitochondrial efficiency and promotes the shift from oxidative phosphorylation to inefficient glycolytic metabolism [120]. This energy deficit manifests fatigue, reduced cognitive function, and impaired cellular repair, symptoms Richard knew all too well.

The immune system dysfunction caused by alcohol is equally profound. Alcohol disrupts the gut microbiome, promoting the growth of harmful bacteria while reducing beneficial species [121]. It damages the intestinal barrier, allowing bacterial products called lipopolysaccharides to enter the bloodstream and trigger systemic inflammation [122]. It impairs the function of immune cells including macrophages, neutrophils, and T lymphocytes, reducing the body's ability to fight infections while paradoxically increasing autoimmune tendencies [123].

Perhaps most notable is alcohol's devastating effect on the lymphatic system. Research has demonstrated that alcohol consumption reduces lymphatic pumping efficiency by up to 60 percent [124]. This impairment persists for 24 to 48 hours after drinking, meaning that someone who drinks several times per week maintains chronic lymphatic insufficiency. Toxins that should be cleared accumulate. Immune cells that should circulate stagnate. The body's drainage system, already challenged by modern sedentary lifestyles, becomes severely compromised.

Chemical Additives, The Invisible Assault

The final member of the Toxic Nine represents perhaps the most insidious threat to human health: the thousands of chemical additives that have infiltrated the modern food supply. In 1950, the average American consumed approximately 2 pounds of synthetic food additives annually. Today, that figure exceeds 140 pounds per person per year, an increase of 7,000 percent [125]. This represents one of the most dramatic changes to human dietary exposure in the history of our species, and the health consequences are only beginning to be understood.

Richard assumed his commitment to 'fresh, locally sourced ingredients' would protect him from chemical additives. He was wrong. His spice blends contained 'natural flavors,' a category that encompasses over 3,000 different chemical compounds [126]. His dairy products contained emulsifiers. His meat was treated with various processing aids. His cooking wines contained sulfites. Even the packaging his ingredients came in leached chemicals into the food. The reality is that avoiding chemical additives entirely has become nearly impossible in the modern food system, even for someone as conscientious as Richard.

The Regulatory Failure

The United States permits approximately 10,000 additives in food, yet the vast majority have never been independently tested for safety [48]. The FDA's 'Generally Recognized as Safe' (GRAS) loophole allows manufacturers to determine on their own that a substance is safe, without any requirement for FDA review or approval [46]. A company can introduce a new chemical additive into the food supply simply by hiring consultants who declare it safe. There is no requirement for long-term testing, no requirement for testing in combination with other additives, and no requirement for testing in vulnerable populations like children.

The contrast with other developed nations is stark. The European Union bans or restricts over 1,300 chemicals that are freely permitted in American food [52]. Substances like potassium bromate (used in bread), BVO (brominated vegetable oil, used in some soft drinks), and various artificial dyes that are banned in Europe as potential carcinogens are found in common American foods. The United States operates under a philosophy that chemicals are safe until proven dangerous, while Europe applies the precautionary principle, requiring proof of safety before approval.

This regulatory failure has turned the American population into unwitting subjects in the largest uncontrolled chemical experiment in human history. We consume combinations of additives that have never been tested together, in quantities that have never been evaluated for long-term safety, beginning in utero and continuing throughout our lives. The chronic disease epidemic we are experiencing may be, in part, the result of this experiment.

Emulsifiers and the Gut Barrier

Among the most damaging categories of food additives are emulsifiers, chemicals used to keep oil and water from separating in processed foods. Common emulsifiers include polysorbate 80, carboxymethylcellulose, and carrageenan, and they are found in everything from ice cream to salad dressings to non-dairy milks. These compounds were assumed to pass through the digestive system without effect. They don't.

Research has revealed that emulsifiers damage the mucus layer that protects the intestinal lining, the crucial barrier that separates the contents of your gut from your bloodstream and immune system [53]. Studies in animals have shown that dietary emulsifiers promote intestinal inflammation, alter the gut microbiome in ways that favor metabolic disease, and increase intestinal permeability [127]. Human studies have confirmed that emulsifier consumption correlates with markers of gut dysfunction and systemic inflammation [128].

The gut mucus layer represents one of the body's most important barriers, and its degradation has far-reaching consequences. When this layer thins, bacteria that should remain confined to the intestinal lumen come into direct contact with immune cells in the gut wall [129]. The result is chronic immune activation, increased intestinal permeability ('leaky gut'), and systemic inflammation that affects every organ system. Emulsifiers essentially dissolve the protective layer between your gut contents and the rest of your body.

Preservatives and Mitochondrial Damage

Chemical preservatives extend shelf life by inhibiting bacterial growth and preventing oxidation, but these same properties often make them toxic to human cells. BHA (butylated hydroxyanisole),

BHT (butylated hydroxytoluene), and TBHQ (tertiary butylhydroquinone) are synthetic antioxidants used in countless processed foods. All three have been shown to damage mitochondrial function in laboratory studies [130].

Sodium benzoate, one of the most common preservatives in beverages and condiments, is particularly concerning. When combined with ascorbic acid (vitamin C), sodium benzoate can form benzene, a known carcinogen [131]. This reaction occurs spontaneously in many products that contain both ingredients. Additionally, sodium benzoate has been shown to damage mitochondrial DNA and impair cellular respiration, contributing to the energy deficiency that characterizes so many modern chronic diseases [132].

The cumulative burden of these preservatives is difficult to assess because they are rarely tested in combination. Someone who consumes processed foods regularly may be exposed to dozens of different preservatives daily, each potentially damaging cells in slightly different ways. The combined effect on mitochondrial function and cellular health remains largely unstudied, but the epidemic of fatigue and metabolic dysfunction in industrialized societies suggests the consequences are severe.

Daniel's Discovery

Daniel was 50 years old, a sales director who traveled constantly for work. He ate most of his meals in airports, hotels, and restaurants. 'I try to make healthy choices,' he told me. 'Grilled chicken instead of fried. Salads instead of burgers. But I feel like I'm getting worse no matter what I do.' His symptoms included persistent fatigue, unexplained weight gain concentrated around his midsection, and a recently diagnosed pre-diabetic blood sugar pattern.

When we analyzed Daniel's diet, the problem became clear. His 'grilled chicken' at restaurants was typically marinated in soybean oil and cooked on a grill brushed with more soybean oil. His 'healthy salads' were drowning in dressings made from seed oils and loaded with emulsifiers and preservatives. His 'light' meals at airports contained as many chemical additives as the fast food he thought he was avoiding. He was making the choices that seemed healthy while still consuming massive amounts of the most damaging substances in the modern food supply.

We developed a travel protocol for Daniel that focused on avoiding the Toxic Nine even in challenging environments. He learned to request olive oil and lemon for salads instead of commercial dressings. He identified restaurants in his regular travel cities that actually cooked with quality fats. He packed his own snacks rather than relying on airport options. Within four months, his energy returned, his weight began normalizing, and his blood sugar improved to fully normal levels. He was still traveling constantly, but he had learned to navigate the modern food landscape safely.

The Hard Truth About Hidden Poisons

Here is what conventional medicine and the food industry do not want you to understand: seed oils, alcohol, and chemical additives are not incidental concerns. They are not minor issues to address after you have fixed the 'real' problems. They are primary drivers of the chronic disease epidemic that is bankrupting our healthcare system and destroying millions of lives.

The food industry has a perverse incentive structure that rewards the use of these substances. Seed oils are dramatically cheaper than traditional fats, adding billions to industry profits. Chemical additives extend shelf life, reducing waste and increasing margins. Alcohol generates over $250 billion annually in sales [133]. These industries spend enormous sums lobbying regulators, funding sympathetic research, and marketing their products as safe or even healthy. The people making you sick are also the people funding the science that claims they're not.

The medical profession has largely failed to recognize these connections. Your doctor, despite years of training, probably knows very little about the health effects of seed oils. They may still be recommending 'moderate' alcohol consumption based on obsolete research. They almost certainly never considered that the chemical additives in your food might be contributing to your symptoms. Medical education focuses on diagnosing and treating disease, not on understanding the environmental factors that create disease in the first place.

The supplement industry often makes things worse by offering 'solutions' that do not address root causes. You can take all the liver support supplements in the world, but if you are still consuming seed oils and alcohol, your liver will continue to deteriorate. You can load up on anti-inflammatory compounds, but if you are still consuming omega-6 fatty acids at 20 times the natural ratio, you will remain chronically inflamed. True healing requires removing the sources of damage, not just trying to counteract them with pills.

Richard's Recovery

Remember Richard from the beginning of this chapter? The restaurant owner couldn't understand why his commitment to fresh, local ingredients wasn't protecting his health. His recovery began when we addressed all three of the final Toxic Nine members simultaneously.

First, we overhauled his restaurant's kitchen. We replaced all seed oils with appropriate cooking fats: olive oil for cold applications, avocado oil for medium heat, coconut oil, and ghee for high-heat cooking. His staff initially resisted the changes, but within weeks they noticed that food actually tasted better. The oils weren't masking the flavor of quality ingredients anymore. Richard estimated the change would cost him an additional $200 per week in oil expenses, but he began marketing the upgrade as a premium feature, and his customers responded enthusiastically.

Second, Richard eliminated alcohol completely. This was the hardest change for him. Wine had been part of his professional identity as a restaurateur. He associated it with sophistication, relaxation, and the European culinary tradition he admired. We reframed his perspective: the great cuisines of the world existed for thousands of years before widespread alcohol consumption became normalized. He could honor food traditions without poisoning himself. By the third month without alcohol, Richard reported deeper sleep, clearer thinking, and energy levels he had not experienced in years.

Third, we systematically eliminated chemical additives from his kitchen. He replaced commercial spice blends with pure spices. He switched to organic dairy products without emulsifiers. He sourced meats that weren't treated with various processing chemicals. He discovered that many 'restaurant supply' products that seemed convenient were actually concentrated sources of additives that his establishment did not need.

Within six months, Richard's transformation was remarkable. His liver enzymes normalized completely. His fatty liver disease, documented on ultrasound, showed significant improvement [134]. His inflammatory markers dropped to normal ranges. He lost 28 of the 35 pounds he had gained. His brain fog cleared so completely that he developed new menu concepts and opened a second location. 'I thought I was eating healthy before,' he told me at his six-month follow-up. 'Now I realize I was eating poison and calling it food. And the crazy thing is, everything tastes better now. The food at my restaurants has never been this good.'

Now that we've completed our examination of the Toxic Nine, the foods and substances that damage the MILA system and drive chronic disease, a natural question arises: what should you eat? The elimination of these harmful substances creates a void that must be filled with nourishing alternatives.

In the next chapter, we will explore the remarkable abundance of whole foods that support rather than damage your body. From clean proteins to healing fats, from nutrient-dense vegetables to properly prepared carbohydrates, you will discover that removing the Toxic Nine does not mean deprivation. It means liberation into a world of real food that satisfies deeply while healing profoundly.

Key Takeaways

The final three members of the Toxic Nine, seed oils, alcohol, and chemical additives, represent the most insidious threats to modern health because they hide in virtually everything we consume.

Seed oils have increased from zero to 20 percent of American calories in just over a century, creating catastrophic omega-6 imbalance and generating toxic aldehydes when heated.

Alcohol, despite decades of false claims about moderate benefits, is classified as a Group 1 carcinogen with no safe level of consumption, damaging every component of the MILA system.

Chemical additives have increased 7,000 percent since 1950, with emulsifiers degrading gut barriers and preservatives damaging mitochondria.

Eliminating these substances requires vigilance but produces remarkable results.

Chapter 5

What to Eat: The Abundance of Whole Foods

Christine sat in my office with tears streaming down her face. At 43, this stay-at-home mother of three had spent the previous six months of her life, learning everything she needed to eliminate from her diet. Sugar. Wheat. Corn. Soy. Dairy. Peanuts. Seed oils. Alcohol. Chemical additives. The Toxic Nine had been the foundation of her family's eating pattern for as long as she could remember. 'I've been up all night,' she said, 'trying to figure out what we can even eat anymore. I feel like you've told me everything is poison. My kids are going to starve. I'm going to starve. There's nothing left.'

Christine's despair was genuine, and I have seen it in countless patients. The first phase of dietary transformation, understanding what to avoid and why, can feel overwhelming. When you realize that the standard American diet is built on a foundation of inflammatory, metabolically damaging substances, it is natural to feel like the rug has been pulled out from under you. Everything you learned about food, everything you have fed your family, everything that seemed normal and safe, suddenly appears dangerous.

But Christine was standing at the threshold of a revelation that would change her relationship with food forever. The Toxic Nine doesn't represent the majority of available foods. It represents a narrow category of industrial products that have displaced real food over the past century. When you eliminate these substances, you don't find yourself in a dietary wasteland. You discover an abundance of whole, nourishing foods that humans have thrived on for thousands of generations, foods that taste better, satisfy more deeply, and heal rather than harm.

'Christine,' I said, 'I haven't told you everything is poison. I've told you that nine categories of industrial food products are poison. That leaves thousands of whole foods that your body was designed to thrive on. Let me show you what real abundance looks like.'

The One-Ingredient Principle

The simplest way to navigate the modern food landscape is to apply what I call the One-Ingredient Principle. If food has only one ingredient, it is almost certainly safe. Chicken is chicken. Broccoli is broccoli. Salmon is salmon. Almonds are almonds. These foods do not require ingredient lists because they are the ingredient. They don't contain hidden sugars, seed oils, or chemical additives because there is nowhere for those substances to hide [135].

This principle immediately clarifies what you can eat. Walk through a grocery store and you will find hundreds of one-ingredient foods: every vegetable in the produce section, every fruit, every cut of fresh meat, every piece of fresh fish, every nut, and seed. These aren't exotic healthy foods. They're the foods that humans ate for hundreds of thousands of years before the industrial food system convinced us that processed products were somehow superior.

The beauty of the One-Ingredient Principle requires no nutritional expertise to apply. You don't need to understand biochemistry or memorize lists of forbidden additives. You simply look at the food and ask: Is this thing what it says it is? Is this chicken just chicken, or does it contain 'chicken product' plus a dozen other ingredients? Is this oatmeal just oats, or does it contain sugar, corn syrup, and artificial flavors? The question answers itself.

When Christine embraced this principle, her anxiety about what to feed her family dissolved almost overnight. She stopped reading ingredient lists because the foods she was buying didn't have ingredient lists. She stopped trying to decode food marketing claims because whole foods do not need marketing. A steak does not need to claim it is 'natural' or 'heart healthy' because it simply is what it is. Her shopping became simpler, her cooking became easier, and her family became healthier.

Clean Protein Sources

Protein forms the structural foundation of the human body. Every cell, every enzyme, every hormone, every neurotransmitter depends on adequate protein intake. When we eliminate the Toxic Nine, we do not eliminate protein. We eliminate the processed, contaminated versions and embrace clean sources that provide what our bodies need without the accompanying damage [136].

Eggs stand as perhaps the most perfect food available to humans. A single egg contains complete protein with all essential amino acids, plus choline for brain health, lutein and zeaxanthin for eye health, vitamins A, D, E, and B12, and a host of minerals [137]. The decades-long fear of eggs based on cholesterol concerns has been thoroughly debunked by modern research. Dietary cholesterol has minimal impact on blood cholesterol for most people, and eggs have been shown to improve cholesterol particle size and overall metabolic markers [138]. Choose pasture-raised eggs, when possible, as chickens that forage on grass and insects produce eggs with significantly higher omega-3 content and a better fatty acid profile [139].

Poultry provides lean, versatile protein that forms a staple of diets worldwide. Chicken and turkey offer excellent protein density with lower fat content than red meat, making them particularly useful for those managing caloric intake. The key is sourcing: look for organic, free-range, or pasture-raised birds that have not been raised on corn and soy with routine antibiotic use [140]. The meat from properly raised poultry contains a healthier fatty acid profile and avoids the accumulation of toxins that concentrate in conventionally raised animals.

Wild-caught fish represents one of the most nutrient-dense protein sources available. Fatty fishlike salmon, mackerel, sardines, and herring provide protein plus substantial omega-3 fatty acids that are essential for brain health, inflammation regulation, and cardiovascular function [141]. These fish also provide vitamin D, selenium, and iodine, nutrients that are difficult to obtain in adequate amounts from other sources. The distinction between wild-caught and farm-raised matters significantly: farmed fish are typically fed corn and soy products, contain higher omega-6 levels, and may accumulate environmental contaminants from crowded aquaculture conditions [142].

Grass-fed beef offers a nutritional profile dramatically different from conventionally raised cattle. Animals that graze on pasture produce meat with higher omega-3 content, more conjugated linoleic acid (CLA), higher levels of antioxidants like vitamin E and beta-carotene, and a significantly better omega-6 to omega-3 ratio [143]. The fear of red meat that has dominated nutritional discourse for decades was largely based on observational studies that failed to distinguish between processed meat and fresh, unprocessed beef. When researchers control for this distinction, the supposed dangers of red meat largely disappear [144].

Wild game provides perhaps the cleanest animal protein available. Venison, elk, bison, and other wild game are naturally free-range, consuming their native diets without human intervention. These meats are typically leaner than domesticated animals with excellent fatty acid profiles and no concerns about antibiotics, hormones, or unnatural feed [145]. For those with access through hunting or specialty markets, wild game represents ancestral eating at its purest.

Pasture-raised pork, while often overlooked, can be an excellent protein source when properly sourced. Pigs raised outdoors on diverse diets including forage, nuts, and natural foods produce meat with better fatty acid composition and no concerns about the concentrated feeding operations that characterize conventional pork production [146]. The key is finding producers who raise pigs in natural conditions rather than the industrial confinement operations that produce the majority of commercial pork.

Tree nuts round out the protein category, providing plant-based protein along with healthy fats, fiber, and numerous micronutrients. Almonds, walnuts, cashews, pecans, macadamia nuts, hazelnuts, and Brazil nuts all offer valuable nutrition [147]. Note that peanuts are not included here because they are legumes, not tree nuts, and are members of the Toxic Nine due to aflatoxin contamination and other concerns. Tree nuts, in contrast, are among the healthiest foods you can eat, associated with reduced cardiovascular disease, better cognitive function, and improved longevity in numerous studies [148].

Lawrence's Protein Transformation

Lawrence was 61, a retired professor who had been vegetarian for thirty years on ethical grounds. He came to me with severe fatigue, muscle wasting, and cognitive decline that had accelerated dramatically in the previous two years. 'I thought I was doing everything right,' he said. 'No meat, lots of soy for protein, whole grains, vegetable oils. I followed the advice perfectly. Now I can barely climb stairs, and my wife says I'm forgetting things.'

Lawrence's case illustrated how well-intentioned dietary choices can go wrong when built on the Toxic Nine foundation. His protein intake had relied heavily on soy products and grain-based meat alternatives, both of which were damaging his health. His 'healthy' vegetable oils were driving inflammation. His whole grains were exposing him to constant gluten and potential glyphosate residues [37].

We had a long conversation about his values and his health. Lawrence wasn't opposed to animal products on nutritional grounds. His concerns were ethical: he did not want to support factory farming or cause unnecessary animal suffering. When I explained that pasture-raised, humanely raised animal products were available, and that his current diet was built on industrial products that caused immense environmental and ethical harm in their production, he agreed to reconsider.

Lawrence began incorporating pasture-raised eggs, wild-caught fish, and small amounts of grass-fed beef from local farms he personally visited. Within four months, his energy returned, his muscle mass began rebuilding, and his cognitive function improved noticeably. His wife reported that he seemed 'like himself again' for the first time in years. He maintained his ethical principles while rebuilding his health, discovering that truly sustainable, humane animal agriculture exists and provides the nutrition his body desperately needed.

Complex Carbohydrates: Energy Without Damage

When we eliminate wheat and corn from the diet, people often assume they must eliminate all carbohydrates. This isn't true. Carbohydrates are not the enemy. Processed, inflammatory, blood-sugar-spiking carbohydrates are the enemy. Whole, complex carbohydrates provide steady energy, essential fiber, and numerous nutrients that support health [149].

Oatmeal stands as an excellent carbohydrate choice when consumed in its whole form. Steel-cut oats and rolled oats provide slow-digesting carbohydrates along with soluble fiber that feeds beneficial gut bacteria and helps regulate cholesterol [150]. Oats contain beta-glucan, a unique fiber that has been shown to improve insulin sensitivity and support immune function [151]. For those sensitive to gluten, certified gluten-free oats are available, as oats do not naturally contain gluten but are often cross-contaminated during processing.

Brown rice offers a whole-grain option that has nourished populations across Asia for millennia. Unlike refined white rice, brown rice retains its bran and germ layers, providing fiber, B vitamins, magnesium, and selenium [152]. The glycemic impact of brown rice is significantly lower than white rice, making it suitable for blood sugar management. Rice is also one of the least allergenic grains, well-tolerated by most people including those with wheat sensitivities.

Quinoa, technically a seed rather than a grain, provides complete protein along with complex carbohydrates. This makes it particularly valuable for those following plant-forward diets who need diverse protein sources [153]. Quinoa also offers excellent amounts of fiber, iron, magnesium, and manganese. Its versatility in cooking, from hot breakfast porridge to cold salads, makes it easy to incorporate into various meals.

Sweet potatoes rank among the most nutritious carbohydrate sources available. Their orange flesh indicates high beta-carotene content, which the body converts to vitamin A [154]. Sweet potatoes also provide vitamin C, potassium, manganese, and various antioxidants including anthocyanins in purple varieties. Despite their name, sweet potatoes have a moderate glycemic index and are well-tolerated by most people managing blood sugar.

White potatoes, often unfairly maligned, can be included in a healthy diet, particularly for those with higher caloric needs such as athletes or those seeking weight gain [155]. Potatoes provide potassium, vitamin C, vitamin B6, and resistant starch when cooled after cooking, which feeds beneficial gut bacteria. The concerns about potatoes relate primarily to the forms in which Americans typically consume them: deep-fried in seed oils or loaded with inflammatory toppings.

Beans and legumes provide carbohydrates along with substantial protein and fiber. Black beans, kidney beans, chickpeas, lentils, and other legumes have nourished human populations for thousands of years [156]. These foods require proper preparation, including soaking and thorough cooking, to reduce anti-nutrients like lectins and phytates. When properly prepared, they offer excellent nutrition and serve as dietary staples in many of the world's healthiest cultures.

Vegetables: The Foundation of the Plate

If there is one category where restriction gives way entirely to abundance, it's vegetables. Virtually all vegetables are not only permitted but encouraged on this protocol. These foods provide fiber, vitamins, minerals, antioxidants, and phytonutrients that support every aspect of MILA function. Vegetables should form the foundation of every lunch and dinner plate, with a target of at least two to three cups per meal [157].

Leafy greens top the list of nutritional powerhouses. Spinach, kale, Swiss chard, collard greens, arugula, and romaine lettuce provide extraordinary nutrient density with minimal calories. These vegetables offer vitamins A, C, K, and folate, along with minerals like iron and calcium. Their chlorophyll content supports detoxification pathways, and their fiber feeds beneficial gut bacteria [158]. Aim to include dark leafy greens daily, varying your choices to obtain a broad spectrum of nutrients.

Cruciferous vegetables deserve special attention for their unique health-promoting compounds. Broccoli, cauliflower, Brussels sprouts, cabbage, and bokchoy contain glucosinolates that the body converts to sulforaphane and other compounds with potent anti-cancer and detoxification-supporting properties [159]. Research has consistently associated regular cruciferous vegetable consumption with reduced cancer risk, improved hormone metabolism, and enhanced liver function [160]. These vegetables should appear in your diet at least several times per week.

Root vegetables provide satisfying, grounding foods that work beautifully in cooler months. Carrots, beets, turnips, parsnips, and radishes offer fiber and unique phytonutrients. Beets are particularly notable for their nitrate content, which supports healthy blood pressure and exercise performance [161]. These vegetables can be roasted, steamed, or eaten raw, providing versatility in meal preparation.

Squash varieties offer both winter and summer options with excellent nutrition. Butternut squash, acorn squash, spaghetti squash, and delicata squash provide complex carbohydrates along with beta-carotene and other antioxidants [162]. Summer squash like zucchini and yellow squash offer lower-carbohydrate alternatives that work well as pasta substitutes or side dishes.

Hydrating vegetables like cucumbers, celery, and bell peppers provide water content along with vitamins and minerals. These vegetables make excellent snacks, providing crunch and satisfaction without significant caloric load [163]. Bell peppers, particularly red and orange varieties, contain remarkably high vitamin C levels, often exceeding citrus fruits ounce to ounce.

Bitter greens including dandelion greens, endive, radicchio, and mustard greens stimulate digestive secretions and support liver function [164]. While their taste takes adjustment for palates accustomed to sweet foods, incorporating small amounts of bitter greens supports digestion and provides unique phytonutrients not found in milder vegetables.

Allium vegetables, the onion family, provide sulfur compounds that support detoxification and immune function. Onions, garlic, leeks, shallots, and chives add flavor to cooking while providing measurable health benefits [165]. Garlic in particular has been associated with cardiovascular benefits, immune support, and antimicrobial properties. These vegetables should be used liberally in cooking.

Fruits: Nature's Sweetness

Fruits provide natural sweetness along with fiber, vitamins, and antioxidants. While we eliminate refined sugars and artificial sweeteners, whole fruits remain part of a healthy diet. The fiber in whole fruit slows sugar absorption, preventing the blood sugar spikes caused by fruit juices or added sugars. Aim for two to three servings of whole fruit daily, prioritizing lower-sugar options while still enjoying the full spectrum of available fruits [166].

Berries represent the optimal fruit choice due to their exceptional antioxidant content and relatively low sugar levels. Blueberries, strawberries, raspberries, and blackberries provide anthocyanins and other polyphenols associated with brain health, cardiovascular protection, and reduced inflammation [167]. Studies have shown that regular berry consumption improves cognitive function and may reduce the risk of age-related cognitive decline [168]. Berries can be consumed fresh, frozen, or added to meals throughout the day.

Citrus fruits offer vitamin C, fiber, and unique flavonoids. Oranges, grapefruits, lemons, and limes provide hydration along with immune-supporting nutrients [169]. The white pith of citrus fruits contains hesperidin and other compounds that support vascular health, so consuming the fruit whole rather than just the juice provides greater benefits.

Stone fruits including peaches, plums, nectarines, and cherries provide seasonal variety with good fiber content. Cherries deserve particular mention for their melatonin content, which can support sleep quality, and their anti-inflammatory properties, which may benefit exercise recovery [170]. These fruits are best consumed fresh and in season when their nutrient content peaks.

Apples and pears offer year-round availability with excellent fiber content, particularly when eaten with the skin [171]. The pectin fiber in apples supports gut health and helps regulate blood sugar. The variety of apples available makes them versatile for different purposes, from eating raw to cooking in savory dishes.

Tropical fruits like mangoes, pineapples, and papayas provide unique enzyme content along with vitamins and flavor. These fruits are higher in sugar than berries but still appropriate in moderate amounts [172]. Papaya contains papain, an enzyme that supports protein digestion. Pineapple provides bromelain, which has anti-inflammatory properties.

Rebecca's Discovery

Rebecca, a 38-year-old graphic designer, had struggled with her weight for years despite what she considered careful eating. When we analyzed her diet, we discovered she was consuming almost no vegetables, relying instead on processed 'low-fat' and 'diet' foods that were loaded with sugar, artificial sweeteners, and chemical additives. 'I hate vegetables,' she said flatly. 'I've hated them since I was a kid. They're bland and boring and I'd rather just eat less of the foods I like.'

Rebecca's aversion to vegetables was common, and it stemmed from a childhood diet that had trained her palate to expect intense sweetness and artificial flavors. Real food, the subtle sweetness of a roasted carrot or the satisfying bitterness of sautéed greens, couldn't compete with the engineered palatability of processed foods [51]. Her taste buds had been hijacked and reclaiming them would require some patience.

We started Rebecca on a gradual transition. Rather than forcing herself to eat steamed broccoli, which she found repulsive, she began with vegetables prepared in ways that added flavor: roasted Brussels sprouts with olive oil and sea salt, cauliflower mashed with garlic and herbs, salads dressed with high-quality olive oil and balsamic vinegar. We added vegetables to dishes she already enjoyed rather than making them the centerpiece of meals she dreaded.

Something remarkable happened over the next three months. As Rebecca eliminated added sugars and artificial flavors from her diet, her taste perception changed. Foods that had seemed bland now tasted complex and satisfying. She started enjoying vegetables she had sworn she hated for thirty years. 'I actually craved a salad yesterday,' she told me with genuine shock. 'I've never craved a vegetable in my life.' Six months later, Rebecca had lost 40 pounds, resolved her chronic digestive issues, and developed what she called 'a totally new relationship with food.' The abundance she discovered wasn't just adequate. It was genuinely pleasurable.

Healthy Fats: Essential for Every Cell

The elimination of industrial seed oils does not mean eliminating fat. Healthy fats are essential for hormone production, brain function, nutrient absorption, and cellular membrane integrity. The key is choosing fats that humans have consumed safely for millennia rather than the industrial products introduced in the past century [173].

Extra virgin olive oil stands as perhaps the healthiest fat available for human consumption. This oil, produced simply by crushing olives, provides monounsaturated fats along with powerful antioxidants including oleocanthal, which has anti-inflammatory properties comparable to ibuprofen [174]. Research consistently associates olive oil consumption with reduced cardiovascular disease, improved cognitive function, and lower all-cause mortality [175]. Use high-quality extra virgin olive oil liberally for dressings, drizzling over finished dishes, and low-to-medium heat cooking.

Avocado oil provides a higher smoke point option for cooking while still offering monounsaturated fats and vitamin E [176]. This oil works well for higher-heat applications like roasting and sautéing. Whole avocados themselves provide excellent nutrition: healthy fats, fiber, potassium, and various vitamins.

Coconut oil offers medium-chain triglycerides (MCTs) that are metabolized differently than other fats, providing quick energy without the insulin response of carbohydrates [177]. Coconut oil is extremely stable for high-heat cooking and adds flavor to dishes where its taste is appropriate. While some have raised concerns about coconut oil's saturated fat content, research has shown that it raises HDL cholesterol and improves other cardiovascular markers in most people [178].

Ghee, or clarified butter, provides the benefits of butter with the milk solids removed, making it suitable for those with dairy sensitivities to the proteins in butter [179]. Ghee has an extremely high smoke point, making it excellent for high-heat cooking. It has been used for thousands of years in Indian cooking and Ayurvedic medicine.

Animal fats from quality sources, including tallow, lard, and duck fat, were dietary staples throughout human history until the vegetable oil revolution [38]. These fats are extremely stable for cooking, provide fat-soluble vitamins, and add exceptional flavor to foods. When sourced from pasture-raised animals, they contain a healthier fatty acid profile than fats from conventionally raised animals.

Putting It All Together: The Abundant Plate

When you combine clean proteins, complex carbohydrates, abundant vegetables, satisfying fruits, and healthy fats, you discover that eliminating the Toxic Nine does not restrict you. It liberates you into a world of real food that our ancestors would have recognized and enjoyed. A typical day might include eggs cooked with vegetables for breakfast, a large salad with wild salmon and olive oil dressing for lunch, and grass-fed beef with roasted vegetables and sweet potato for dinner. Snacks might include tree nuts, fresh fruit, or vegetables with guacamole. This is not deprivation. This is abundance.

The variety available within whole foods far exceeds what the processed food industry offers. Consider vegetables alone: there are hundreds of varieties of edible plants, each with unique flavors, textures, and nutritional profiles. Add the variety of clean proteins, the different preparations possible with healthy fats, the seasonal changes in available fruits, and you have virtually unlimited options for delicious, satisfying meals [180].

Christine discovered this abundance over the following months. What began as despair transformed into enthusiasm as she explored new foods and cooking methods. Her children, initially resistant, adapted faster than she expected when they weren't constantly bombarded by hyper-palatable processed foods. The meals she prepared became family events rather than battles. She spent less money on food because she was buying ingredients rather than products. And most importantly, her family's health has transformed.

Christine's Transformation

Six months after her tearful declaration that there was nothing left to eat, Christine returned to my office a different person. She had lost 25 pounds without ever counting calories. Her chronic joint pain had resolved. Her afternoon energy crashes were gone. Her two older children, previously diagnosed with ADHD, were performing better in school without any change in their medication. Her youngest, who had suffered from chronic eczema since infancy, had clear skin for the first time [181].

'I can't believe I was so scared,' she told me. 'The food we eat now is so much better than what we ate before. The kids don't even ask for the old stuff anymore. Last week my 10-year-old said she felt bad for her friends who eat fake food at lunch. She's proud of what she eats. I never thought that would happen.'

Christine's transformation illustrates the central truth of this chapter: eliminating the Toxic Nine does not leave you in dietary poverty. It opens the door to a way of eating that is more satisfying, more flavorful, and infinitely more nourishing than the industrial diet it replaces. The abundance of whole foods is not just adequate. It is extraordinary.

Understanding what to eat is only half the equation. The next crucial question is how much and when.

In the following chapter, we will explore the daily structure that optimizes MILA function: personalized portions based on your body size and activity level, the science of meal timing, and the powerful practice of 16:8 intermittent fasting.

These practical tools transform theoretical knowledge into a sustainable daily pattern that supports healing and long-term health. The abundance you have discovered needs structure to become sustainable, and that structure awaits.

Key Takeaways

The elimination of the Toxic Nine does not create dietary restrictions but rather opens access to the abundance of whole, one-ingredient foods that humans thrived on for millennia.

Clean proteins from pasture-raised eggs, wild-caught fish, grass-fed beef, and tree nuts provide complete nutrition without inflammatory burden.

Complex carbohydrates from oats, rice, quinoa, sweet potatoes, and legumes offer steady energy without blood sugar disruption.

Vegetables form the unlimited foundation of every plate, providing fiber, vitamins, minerals, and phytonutrients.

Fruits offer natural sweetness with fiber-bound nutrients.

Healthy fats from olive oil, avocado, coconut, and animal sources support every cellular function.

This is liberation, not deprivation.

Chapter 6

The Daily Structure: Portions, Timing, and 16:8 Fasting.

Steven's Metabolic Rollercoaster

Steven was 47 years old, a successful financial advisor who made his living analyzing numbers and managing risks. Yet when it came to his own body, he had lost all control. Every afternoon around 2 PM, his energy crashed so severely that he needed three cups of coffee just to make it through client meetings. By 4 PM, the hunger was unbearable, driving him to the vending machine for whatever could quiet the gnawing in his stomach.

'I know I'm eating too much,' Steven admitted during our first consultation. 'But I feel like I have no choice. Hunger is overwhelming. If I try to eat less at lunch, I can't function in the afternoon. If I skip breakfast, I'm shaky and irritable by 10 AM. My body seems to demand constant feeding, and I don't understand why.'

Steven's blood work revealed the answer. His fasting glucose was 118, just two points below the diabetic threshold. His fasting insulin was elevated at 22, indicating that his cells were becoming resistant to insulin's message. His triglycerides were high, his HDL cholesterol was low, and his hemoglobin A1c suggested he'd been running elevated blood sugars for months. Steven was on a blood sugar rollercoaster [182].

The problem was not weakness or lack of willpower; the problem was that Steven had never been taught how to eat. Not what to eat, but how much and when. His meals were randomly timed, inconsistently sized, and designed to spike blood sugar as rapidly as possible. Breaking this cycle would require restructuring his entire relationship with eating.

Understanding Your Portions

We have already learned what you put in your body is extremely important. But how much you put in, and when, is just as important.

Portion size varies dramatically based on body weight, activity level, metabolic health, and personal goals. The charts below provide personalized guidance based on your current weight and activity level, specifying actual amounts of food in practical measurements.

Personalized Portion Calculator

To determine your specific portions for each meal, use the following charts based on your weight, activity level, and goals. These portions are designed to provide optimal nutrition while supporting your health objectives.

Understanding What the Charts Account For

The charts below are designed around the primary factors that determine your caloric and macronutrient needs:

Weight: Larger bodies require more energy and nutrients to function. The weight ranges in the left column provide appropriate base portions that scale with body size.

Activity Level: Physical activity dramatically increases energy expenditure and nutrient requirements, particularly for carbohydrates which fuel muscle activity. Athletes and highly active individuals need substantially more carbohydrates to maintain performance and recovery. This is why the columns across the top vary so much—a sedentary 160lb person needs very different portions than an athletic 160lb person. Be honest with yourself — most people overestimate their activity:

- Sedentary: Little to no exercise, desk job, minimal daily movement
- Light Active: Light exercise or sports 1-3 days per week
- Moderate: Moderate exercise or sports 3-5 days per week

- Heavy: Hard exercise or sports 6-7 days per week
- Athlete: Very intense exercise daily, physical labor job, or competitive athlete training

Sex Considerations: While not explicitly separated in the charts, sex differences are accounted for through weight ranges. Women typically fall into lower weight ranges with corresponding lower portions, while men typically fall into higher ranges. The activity multipliers further personalized needs based on your individual lifestyle.

Age Adjustments: Older adults (50+) with the same weight and activity level may find they do better at the lower end of their prescribed range, while younger adults (18-30) may need the higher end or even slightly more. Metabolism naturally slows with age, so adjust within your range based on your results and energy levels.

How to Use the Portion Charts

The following charts will show you exactly how much protein, carbohydrates, vegetables, fruit, and nuts to eat at each meal. Here is how to use them:

- Find your weight range in the left column of each chart
- Identify your activity level across the top row
- Read the portions for Breakfast (B), Lunch (L), and Dinner (D)

- Apply goal modifiers if you're specifically targeting weight loss or gain (noted below each chart)
- Measure portions using measuring cups and/or a food scale until you can estimate accurately by sight

Important: The protein chart shows ounces of cooked protein (weight after cooking). The carbohydrate chart shows cups of cooked grains, beans, or potatoes (measure after cooking).

Raw vs. Cooked Conversions

Protein (eggs, meat, poultry, fish): Loses about 25% weight during cooking. To get your cooked target, buy/cook about 33% more raw weight.

- Example: For 6 oz cooked chicken, start with 8 oz raw
- Simple rule: Raw weight × 0.75 = Cooked weight

Grains (rice, quinoa, oats): Roughly triple in volume when cooked.

- Example: ⅓ cup dry rice → 1 cup cooked rice
- Simple rule: Divide your cooked target by 3 to get dry amount

Beans (dried): Roughly triple in volume when cooked.

- Example: ⅓ cup dry beans → 1 cup cooked beans
- Or use canned: 1 cup canned (drained) = 1 cup cooked

Sweet potatoes/white potatoes: Minimal change in weight when baked or steamed.

- Simple rule: 1 cup raw cubed ≈ 1 cup cooked cubed

Goal Modifiers:

- Weight Loss: Reduce all carb amounts by ¼ cup from the chart
- Weight Gain: Add white potatoes to meals and increase amount of carbs by ¼ cup

PROTEIN (oz per meal cooked)

Weight Range	Sedentary	Light Active	Moderate	Heavy	Athlete
100-120 lbs	B:2.5 L:3 D:3	B:3 L:3.5 D:3.5	B:3 L:4 D:4	B:3.5 L:4.5 D:4.5	B:4 L:5 D:5
121-140 lbs	B:3 L:3.5 D:3.5	B:3.5 L:4 D:4	B:3.5 L:4.5 D:4.5	B:4 L:5 D:5	B:4.5 L:5.5 D:5.5
141-160 lbs	B:3.5 L:4 D:4	B:4 L:4.5 D:4.5	B:4 L:5 D:5	B:4.5 L:5.5 D:5.5	B:5 L:6 D:6
161-180 lbs	B:4 L:4.5 D:4.5	B:4.5 L:5 D:5	B:4.5 L:5.5 D:5.5	B:5 L:6 D:6	B:5.5 L:6.5 D:6.5
181-200 lbs	B:4.5 L:5 D:5	B:5 L:5.5 D:5.5	B:5 L:6 D:6	B:5.5 L:6.5 D:6.5	B:6 L:7 D:7
201-220 lbs	B:5 L:5.5 D:5.5	B:5.5 L:6 D:6	B:5.5 L:6.5 D:6.5	B:6 L:7 D:7	B:6.5 L:7.5 D:7.5
221-240 lbs	B:5.5 L:6 D:6	B:6 L:6.5 D:6.5	B:6 L:7 D:7	B:6.5 L:7.5 D:7.5	B:7 L:8 D:8
240+ lbs	B:6 L:6.5 D:6.5	B:6.5 L:7 D:7	B:6.5 L:7.5 D:7.5	B:7 L:8 D:8	B:7.5 L:9 D:9

B=Breakfast, L=Lunch, D=Dinner

CARBS (cups per meal cooked)

Weight Range	Sedentary	Light Active	Moderate	Heavy	Athlete
100-120 lbs	B:⅓ L:⅓ D:⅓	B:½ L:½ D:½	B:½ L:½ D:½	B:¾ L:¾ D:¾	B:¾ L:1 D:1
121-140 lbs	B:⅓ L:⅓ D:⅓	B:½ L:½ D:½	B:½ L:¾ D:¾	B:¾ L:¾ D:¾	B:1 L:1 D:1
141-160 lbs	B:½ L:½ D:½	B:½ L:¾ D:¾	B:¾ L:¾ D:¾	B:¾ L:1 D:1	B:1 L:1.25 D:1.25
161-180 lbs	B:½ L:½ D:½	B:¾ L:¾ D:¾	B:¾ L:¾ D:¾	B:1 L:1 D:1	B:1.25 L:1.5 D:1.5
181-200 lbs	B:½ L:¾ D:¾	B:¾ L:¾ D:¾	B:¾ L:1 D:1	B:1 L:1.25 D:1.25	B:1.5 L:1.5 D:1.5
201-220 lbs	B:¾ L:¾ D:¾	B:¾ L:1 D:1	B:1 L:1 D:1	B:1.25 L:1.5 D:1.5	B:1.5 L:1.75 D:1.75
221-240 lbs	B:¾ L:¾ D:¾	B:1 L:1 D:1	B:1 L:1.25 D:1.25	B:1.5 L:1.5 D:1.5	B:1.75 L:2 D:2
240+ lbs	B:¾ L:1 D:1	B:1 L:1 D:1	B:1.25 L:1.25 D:1.25	B:1.5 L:1.75 D:1.75	B:2 L:2 D:2

VEGETABLES (cups per meal)

Activity Level	Per Meal (Lunch & Dinner)	Daily Minimum
All levels	2-3 cups	4-6 cups total

Note: Vegetables are unlimited—these are minimums. The more vegetables, the better.

FRUIT (cups per serving)

Goal	Per Serving (Breakfast & Afternoon Snack)	Daily Total
Weight Loss	1 cup	2 cups
Maintenance	1-1.5 cups	2-3 cups
Weight Gain/Athlete	1.5-2 cups	3-4 cups

Berries are preferred due to their superior antioxidant content and lower sugar impact.

NUTS (oz for mid-morning snack)

Weight Range	Amount (oz)
100-140 lbs	1 oz
141-180 lbs	1.5 oz
181-220 lbs	2 oz
221+ lbs	2.5 oz

Approximately: 1 oz = small handful, 1.5 oz = generous handful, 2 oz = large handful

Important Note on Portion Sizes

These portions may initially appear larger than what you are accustomed to eating, but this is intentional and based on sound metabolic science. When eating in this thermic, protein-rich manner combined with high-fiber whole foods, your body utilizes significantly more calories for digestion, absorption, and metabolism—a process known as the thermic effect of food (TEF).

Protein requires 20-30% of its calories just to be processed, compared to only 5-10% for carbohydrates and 0-3% for fats. Additionally, the high fiber content from vegetables, fruits, and whole grains creates bulk and promotes satiety without adding significant absorbable calories, as much of the fiber passes through undigested while feeding beneficial gut bacteria.

The result is that you can consume a much higher volume of food without feeling overly full or gaining unwanted weight—in fact, most patients lose fat while building or maintaining muscle mass on these portions. Your body becomes more metabolically active, burning more calories at rest while being properly nourished.

The Science of Meal Timing

For most of human history, the question of when to eat was determined by food availability rather than personal choice. Our ancestors ate when food was available and fasted when it wasn't.

This intermittent pattern was not a hardship but rather the normal condition under which human metabolism evolved.

Modern life has eliminated natural periods of fasting. Most Americans eat from the moment they wake until they fall asleep, consuming an average of 15 hours worth of meals and snacks daily. The constant influx of calories keeps insulin perpetually elevated and never allows the body to shift into the fat-burning, repair-promoting fasted state that our physiology requires.

When insulin remains elevated, cells become progressively resistant to its signal, requiring ever-higher levels to achieve the same glucose-lowering effect. This insulin resistance promotes fat storage, drives inflammation, disrupts hormone balance, and creates the blood sugar instability that Steven experienced.

Perhaps most significantly, constant feeding prevents autophagy, the cellular self-cleaning process that removes damaged proteins and dysfunctional mitochondria. When we never fast, cellular debris accumulates, mitochondrial function declines, and the terrain becomes increasingly toxic.

The 16:8 Intermittent Fasting Protocol

The 16:8 intermittent fasting protocol compresses all eating into an 8-hour window and fasts for the remaining 16 hours. This pattern aligns with human evolutionary biology, provides adequate nutrition during the eating window, and allows sufficient fasting time to activate repair mechanisms.

For most people, this means eating, for example, between approximately 6 AM to 2 PM, 8 AM and 4 PM, or noon and 8 PM. The eating window can be adjusted: someone who prefers breakfast might eat from 8 AM to 4 PM, while someone with evening commitments might eat from 2 PM to 10 PM. The specific timing matters less than maintaining 16 hours of fasting.

During the fasting window, plain water should be consumed liberally. Black coffee is acceptable and may enhance some fasting benefits. Unsweetened tea is also appropriate. What must be avoided is anything with calories, artificial sweeteners, or flavors that trigger an insulin response.

The Biological Benefits of Fasting

Insulin sensitivity improves dramatically when the body experiences regular periods without food. Studies show that time-restricted eating improves insulin sensitivity independent of calorie intake or weight loss.

Autophagy activation occurs when insulin drops and nutrients become scarce. During this cellular housekeeping process, the body breaks down damaged proteins, clears dysfunctional mitochondria, and recycles cellular components. The 16-hour fasting window provides sufficient time for meaningful autophagy activation.

Growth hormone elevation during fasting preserves lean muscle mass while burning fat. Studies show that 24-hour fasting can increase growth hormone by up to 2000 percent in men and 1300 percent in women. While a 16-hour fast produces more modest increases, the cumulative effect supports muscle maintenance and tissue repair.

Fat oxidation increases as the body shifts from burning glucose to burning stored fat. After approximately 12 hours of fasting, glycogen stores deplete and the body relies on fat for fuel. This metabolic flexibility is a hallmark of metabolic health.

Inflammation decreases as the gut immune system gets a daily rest period during fasting. Inflammatory markers typically improve with intermittent fasting, contributing to reduced chronic disease risk.

Putting Portions and Timing Together

Below is an outline of how the portions above would be timed in a 16:8 fasting day.

Breakfast (Hour 0): Protein + Carbohydrate + Fruit

Starting the day with protein, complex carbohydrates, and fruit provides sustained energy, stabilizes blood sugar, and prevents mid-morning crashes.

Protein provides amino acids for muscle maintenance and satiety. The complex carbohydrate provides sustained energy. The fruit provides quick-absorbing micronutrients, fiber, and antioxidants to start the day.

Snack (Hour 2): Nuts

A measured portion of tree nuts (using the chart above) provides healthy fats, protein, fiber, and minerals to maintain energy and satiety until lunch. This prevents blood sugar crashes and the temptation to reach for processed snacks.

Lunch (Hour 4): Protein + Carbohydrate + Vegetables.

The midday meal should be substantial, providing energy for the afternoon while emphasizing vegetables.

The vegetable component should be generous—at least half the plate by volume. This ensures adequate fiber, micronutrient intake, and satiety with minimal calories.

Snack (Hour 6): Fruit

Whole fruit (per the chart based on your goals) provides natural sugars for an energy boost along with fiber, vitamins, and hydration. This helps maintain energy through the late afternoon and prevents excessive hunger at dinner.

Dinner (Hour 8): Protein + Carbohydrate + Vegetables

The evening meal follows the same structure as lunch, with an emphasis on earlier eating, when possible, to allow digestion before sleep.

Below is a chart outlining a sample of a standard day. Insert your portion sizes based on the charts above.

Sample Meal Plan

Breakfast - Hour 0	Protein	Carb	Veggies	Fruit	Water
Snack - Hour 2	Nuts				Water
Lunch - Hour 4	Protein	Carb	Veggies		Water
Snack - Hour 6				Fruit	Water
Dinner - Hour 8	Protein	Carb	Veggies		Water

Seasoning and Flavor

Food should be delicious and satisfying, not bland and boring. Liberal use of herbs and spices is encouraged, as many have anti-inflammatory and health-promoting properties:

- Herbs: Basil, cilantro, parsley, rosemary, thyme, oregano, sage, mint, and dill all provide flavor and beneficial compounds

- Spices: Turmeric, ginger, cinnamon, black pepper, cumin, coriander, paprika, and cayenne provide not only flavor but anti-inflammatory and metabolic benefits

- Garlic and onions: Fundamental flavoring agents with proven health benefits
- Citrus: Lemon and lime juice provide acidity and brightness without adding sugar
- Vinegars: Apple cider vinegar, balsamic vinegar, and red wine vinegar add flavor and may improve blood sugar control

Critical Caveat

Many commercial spice blends and seasonings contain hidden sugars, seed oils, MSG, and other additives. Always read ingredient labels on any pre-mixed seasonings. When in doubt, buy individual spices and herbs and mix your own blends.

Why This Protocol Works

This eating pattern succeeds where countless diets fail because it addresses the root causes of metabolic dysfunction rather than simply restricting calories:

- Eliminates inflammatory foods: By removing the Toxic 9, systemic inflammation decreases, allowing the body to heal
- Stabilizes blood sugar: The combination of protein, fiber-rich complex carbohydrates, and healthy fats prevents the

blood sugar roller coaster that drives hunger and fat storage

- Supports the gut microbiome: High fiber intake from vegetables, fruits, beans, and whole grains feeds beneficial bacteria
- Provides complete nutrition: Unlike restrictive diets that eliminate entire food groups, this protocol includes all essential nutrients from whole food sources
- Naturally controls portions: Whole foods high in protein and fiber provide satiety, making calorie restriction unnecessary so that your appetite self-regulates
- Sustainable long-term: Because no foods are fundamentally 'forbidden' (only processed versions are avoided), and the variety is substantial, people can follow this approach indefinitely
- Addresses MILA system health: By eliminating mitochondrial toxins, supporting immune function through gut health, and reducing lymphatic congestion through anti-inflammatory eating, this protocol supports the body's fundamental systems

Expected Outcomes

When followed consistently, patients typically experience:

- Weight loss: 1-2 pounds per week for those needing to lose weight, without hunger or deprivation
- Improved energy: Stable blood sugar means consistent energy throughout the day, no afternoon crashes [183]
- Reduced inflammation: Joint pain, headaches, and inflammatory conditions often improve dramatically [184]
- Better digestion: Bloating, gas, and digestive discomfort typically resolve as the gut heals [185]
- Normalized blood sugar: Pre-diabetes often reverses; type 2 diabetes improves significantly and medication may be reduced [186]
- Improved cardiovascular markers: Cholesterol, triglycerides, and blood pressure typically improve [187]
- Mental clarity: Many patients report improved focus, mood, and cognitive function [188]
- Better sleep: Without blood sugar fluctuations and inflammatory burden, sleep quality often improves [189]
- Reduced medication needs: As health improves, many patients can reduce or eliminate medications for blood pressure, diabetes, acid reflux, and other conditions (always under physician supervision) [190]

This Isn't a Diet—It's a Return to Normal

The most important realization for patients is that this is not some extreme or restrictive 'diet'—it is simply eating real food the way humans ate for thousands of years before industrial food processing [62]. The Blue Zones prove that this approach supports health and longevity [59]. Our grandparents' generation ate this way by default because processed foods had not been invented yet [135].

What seems 'restrictive' is only the removal of foods that should not be called 'food' at all—industrial products made in factories from chemical ingredients that did not exist in nature until recently [191]. When patients shift their perspective from 'giving up' processed foods to 'gaining' real health, the transition becomes much easier.

The human body has extraordinary capacity to heal when given the right raw materials and freed from constant assault by inflammatory substances. This protocol provides exactly that opportunity.

Transitioning to the Protocol

Begin by gradually extending your overnight fast. If you currently eat from 7 AM to 10 PM, start by pushing breakfast to 8 AM, then 9 AM, then 10 AM, until you reach your target eating window.

Stay well hydrated during the fasting window. When hunger arises, drink a full glass of water and wait 20 minutes. Plan your eating window meals in advance. Be patient with yourself; some people adapt within days while others need several weeks.

Steven's Transformation

Remember Steven? We started him on a 14-hour fasting window and gradually extended to 16 hours. We calculated his portions based on his 215 pounds and Sedentary activity level. The first week was difficult, but by week three, his morning hunger diminished dramatically.

Steven's three-month results were remarkable. His fasting glucose dropped from 118 to 94. His fasting insulin normalized. His triglycerides dropped by 60 percent. He lost 28 pounds without feeling deprived. 'I finally understand what it feels like to have a normal relationship with food,' he said. 'I'm not constantly thinking about my next meal. I have control for the first time in decades.'

You now have the complete framework for what to eat, how much to eat, and when to eat. But theoretical knowledge must translate into real-world practice. Life happens in restaurants, at social gatherings, and during travel.

In the next chapter, we will explore practical strategies for navigating these challenges: how to eat out while maintaining the protocol, how to handle social pressure, and how to maintain progress when the optimal choice isn't available.

Key Takeaways

Portions must be individualized based on body weight and activity level, with charts provided offering practical guidance for protein, carbohydrates, vegetables, fruits, and nuts.

The 16:8 intermittent fasting protocol compresses eating into an eight-hour window while fasting for sixteen hours, activating powerful metabolic benefits including improved insulin sensitivity, autophagy activation, growth hormone elevation, enhanced fat oxidation, and reduced inflammation.

The transition to time-restricted eating may require several weeks of gradual adaptation, but the metabolic flexibility that develops eliminates blood sugar crashes, constant hunger, and energy instability.

Structure creates freedom, not restriction.

CHAPTER 7

Real-World Navigation

Karen walked into my office carrying a leather briefcase stuffed with restaurant receipts, airline itineraries, and a food journal that read like a confession. At 49, this pharmaceutical sales representative had spent the last eight months trying to follow the protocol while logging over 100,000 miles in the air, entertaining physicians at upscale restaurants, and navigating hotel breakfasts that seemed designed to sabotage her progress. 'I understand science,' she said, her voice tight with frustration. 'I know what I'm supposed to eat. But my life doesn't happen in a controlled kitchen. It happens in airport terminals, client dinners, and conference buffets. Every week feels like starting over.'

Her medical chart told a familiar story: chronic fatigue that had been building for years. Joint pain that her rheumatologist attributed to 'just getting older.' Brain fog that made her once-sharp memory unreliable. She had gained forty pounds over the past decade despite exercising religiously during her increasingly rare days at home. Her fasting blood sugar had crept into pre-diabetic territory. Her inflammatory markers were elevated. And despite her determination to heal through nutrition, her traveling lifestyle seemed to make compliance impossible.

'I've tried everything,' Karen continued. 'I pack protein bars, but they all contain something on the avoid list. I order salads at restaurants, but they come drenched in seed oil dressings. I skip the breadbasket, then find myself ravenous at midnight in my hotel room, ordering room service pizza because it's the only thing available. I feel like I'm failing constantly.'

What Karen did not realize, and what so many patients in similar situations fail to understand, is that navigating real-world eating isn't about willpower. It is about strategy. The modern food environment is specifically designed to make healthy eating difficult, with inflammatory ingredients hidden in almost everything and convenience foods engineered to be irresistible [192]. Success requires not just knowing what to eat, but developing systems, scripts, and strategies that work in the chaos of real life.

The Real-World Challenge

The dietary principles outlined in previous chapters are straightforward when you are eating at home, with complete control over ingredients. You can read every label. You can choose your cooking oils. You can prepare exactly what your body needs. But life doesn't happen entirely in your kitchen. Social obligations, professional demands, travel, and simple convenience all create situations where perfect compliance becomes impossible [193].

This reality trips up countless patients. They understand the science. They are motivated to heal. But the gap between knowing what to eat and successfully eating it in the real world defeats them. They experience a restaurant meal filled with hidden seed oils, feel the inflammatory response in their body the next day, and conclude that the protocol 'doesn't work for them,' or that their lifestyle makes compliance impossible.

The truth is that imperfect compliance, with the right strategy, produces far better results than perfect compliance that lasts only a few days, before real-world pressures cause complete abandonment. The goal isn't perfection; it is sustainable progress. Achieving sustainable progress requires practical strategies for every situation life throws at you [194].

Mastering Restaurant Dining

Restaurant meals present specific challenges. You can't see the ingredients. You don't control the cooking methods. And social pressure often discourages 'difficult' requests. Yet with the right approach, restaurant dining can be navigated successfully without becoming a person who interrogates servers and makes everyone uncomfortable [195].

The Universal Ordering Strategy

Regardless of cuisine type, certain patterns work consistently:

Grilled, baked, or broiled proteins form your foundation. Request that fish, chicken, or steak be prepared dry or with olive oil, ghee, lard, or tallow rather than 'vegetable oil,' which is restaurant code for seed oils. Most restaurants accommodate this request without difficulty because olive oil and animal grease are standard kitchen staples [196].

Steamed, roasted, or grilled vegetables provide your fiber and micronutrients. Avoid anything described as 'crispy' or 'fried,' which guarantees seed oil exposure. Request vegetables without sauce or ask for sauce on the side so you can control the amount.

Side salads with olive oil and vinegar, requested separately, allow you to dress your own greens. House dressings almost universally contain seed oils, sugar, and often soy. By asking for oil and vinegar or lemon wedges, you eliminate this hidden source of inflammation [197].

Baked potatoes or sweet potatoes, when available, provide clean carbohydrates. Request them plain or with olive oil, rather than butter, if you're avoiding dairy. Rice, while not ideal for every meal, represents a cleaner carbohydrate option than bread or pasta when eating out.

Simple Scripts That Work

Having practiced phrases ready reduces anxiety and increases success. These scripts communicate your needs without requiring extensive explanation:

'Can the salmon be prepared dry, or with olive oil, instead of vegetable oil?' This simple request addresses seed oil exposure without requiring you to explain your entire dietary philosophy. Most servers simply say yes [198].

'I'll have grilled chicken with steamed vegetables and a side salad. Oil and vinegar on the side, please.' This orders a complete, compliant meal in a single sentence.

'Could I substitute the pasta for a baked potato?' or 'Can I get vegetables instead of rice?' Simple substitution requests are routine for restaurants.

'No breadbasket for the table, thanks.' Eliminating temptation is easier than resisting it. This phrase, delivered casually, prevents the willpower battle that bread baskets create.

If pressed for reasons, 'I'm focusing on protein and vegetables for health reasons' satisfies most curiosity without inviting debate or requiring detailed explanation [199].

Cuisine-Specific Navigation

Different cuisines present different challenges and opportunities:

Steakhouses represent the easiest option. Steak or fish, steamed vegetables, side salad with oil and vinegar. The primary caution is avoiding butter/dairy additions by requesting olive oil for cooking [200]. These restaurants expect customization requests and accommodate them readily.

Mexican restaurants can work well with modifications. Fajitas without tortillas, served over lettuce, provide protein and vegetables. Guacamole and pico de gallo are typically safe. The challenges are seed oils used in cooking, cheese on everything, and the temptation of chips and margaritas. Specify 'no cheese, no sour cream' and ask about cooking oils [201].

Italian restaurants require avoiding their signature offerings, pasta, and bread, but grilled fish or chicken with vegetables works well. Request olive oil for preparation, which Italian restaurants typically have in abundance. Avoid anything 'parmigiana' (breaded and cheesed) or cream-based [202].

Asian cuisines (Chinese, Thai, Japanese) present the greatest challenges due to high seed oil use, soy sauce in everything, and cornstarch thickeners. At Japanese restaurants, sashimi (plain raw fish) is ideal. At Chinese restaurants, steamed dishes with sauce on the side offer the best options. Thai curries made with coconut milk can work if no soy sauce is added. Request 'no MSG' and be aware that compliance will be imperfect [203].

Indian restaurants offer tandoori dishes (grilled in a clay oven) as your safest choice. Avoid naan, cream-based curries, and dishes with unknown sauces. Many vegetable sides are prepared with healthier fats but ask about ghee versus vegetable oil [204].

The Road Warrior's Dilemma

Thomas, 56, drove a truck for a regional delivery company. His 'office' was the cab of an eighteen-wheeler, his 'lunchroom' was whatever exit had a truck stop, and his eating schedule was dictated by delivery windows rather than hunger. When he first came to see me, his blood pressure required three medications to control, his weight had climbed to 290 pounds, and his doctor had warned him that diabetes was inevitable within a year or two.

'Doc, I know what you're going to tell me,' he said. 'Eat healthy, lose weight. But have you seen what's available at truck stops? It's fried everything or nothing. I can't exactly pack a salad that'll stay fresh for a three-day haul.'

Thomas's situation seemed impossible, but it was not. It required rethinking the entire approach to food-on-the-road.

Travel and On-the-Road Eating

Travel, whether by car, truck, or airplane, creates unique challenges. Limited options, unpredictable schedules, and the disruption of normal routines all conspire against healthy eating. Yet travel is also where strategy matters most because the default options are almost universally inflammatory [205].

The Preparation Principle

The single most important factor in successful travel eating is preparation. When you wait until you are hungry and searching for food, your brain defaults to seeking the quickest, highest-calorie option available, an evolutionary survival mechanism that works against you in modern food environments [206].

For car and truck travel, a cooler transforms everything. Pack pre-cooked chicken, hard-boiled eggs, cut vegetables, pre-portioned nuts, and whole fruit. What seems like extra effort before departure prevents countless poor decisions during the trip. The few minutes spent preparing saves hours of regret and days of inflammatory recovery [207].

For air travel, TSA allows solid foods through security. Pre-cooked proteins, vegetables, fruit, and nuts all travel well. Avoid anything with liquid sauces that might be confiscated. A small, insulated bag keeps food fresh for flights of reasonable length.

Research your destination before arrival. Identify restaurants near your hotel that can accommodate your needs. Note the location of grocery stores where you can stock your hotel room refrigerator with compliant foods. This five minutes of research prevents desperate decisions later.

Airport and Hotel Survival

Airports have improved considerably in recent years, but most options remain problematic. The best airport strategy remains bringing your own food, but when that's not possible:

Look for restaurants with grilled options rather than fast food. Many airports now have sit-down restaurants serving grilled proteins and salads. Yes, they cost more and take longer. Your health is worth both.

Convenience stores and newsstands sell acceptable emergency options: plain nuts (check for added oils), whole fruit, water. These aren't ideal meals, but they prevent worse choices.

Hotel breakfasts typically offer eggs, which can be ordered scrambled or as an omelet with vegetables. Request preparation with olive oil rather than 'spray' (seed oil). Fresh fruit is usually available. Skip pastries, cereals, and juice (liquid sugar).

Hotel rooms with refrigerators allow you to shop on arrival. A quick grocery store visit stocks you with hard-boiled eggs, pre-cooked chicken, cut vegetables, nuts, and fruit that provide several days of compliant eating regardless of what meetings or events throw at you.

Fast Food as Last Resort

Fast food should be a true last resort, not a regular strategy. But when you're on an unfamiliar highway at 10 PM and the only options are fast food chains, some choices are dramatically better than others [208].

Chipotle and similar fast-casual restaurants offer burrito bowls that can be customized to compliance: lettuce base, protein (chicken, steak, or carnitas), fajita vegetables, guacamole, and pico de gallo. Skip the rice, beans, cheese, and sour cream. This isn't perfect, as cooking oils remain a concern, but it is dramatically better than most alternatives [209].

At traditional fast-food restaurants, any burger without the bun represents your best option. Request no cheese and no mayo. Most toppings (lettuce, tomato, onion, pickles, mustard) are acceptable. Some restaurants offer lettuce wraps as an alternative to buns [210].

Grilled chicken options, when available, beat fried alternatives. Grilled nuggets or grilled chicken sandwiches without the bun provide protein without the inflammatory seed oil coating of fried foods.

What to always avoid at fast food: anything fried (seed oils and breading), buns and wraps (wheat and often seed oils), sauces and dressings (sugar, seed oils, soy), cheese, and all beverages except water, black coffee, or unsweetened tea.

Gas Station Emergency Protocol

Sometimes the only option is a gas station convenience store. This is survival mode, not optimal eating, but even here some choices prevent disaster.

Acceptable emergency options include plain nuts (almonds, cashews, walnuts), checking ingredients for added oils. Fresh fruit if available, though selection is often limited. Some convenience stores now carry hard-boiled eggs. Beef jerky can work but check ingredients carefully as many contain sugar and soy. Plain water, black coffee, or unsweetened tea.

Everything else in a gas station should be considered off-limits: chips, candy, pastries, hot dogs, sodas, energy drinks, and the 'trail mix' that's actually chocolate and sugar-coated candy masquerading as health food.

The best gas station strategy is never needing one. A cooler packed before departure, even a small soft-sided cooler for day trips, eliminates the desperation that leads to poor choices [211].

Navigating Social Situations

Food and social connection are deeply intertwined in human culture. Meals mark celebrations, cement business relationships, and provide the context for family bonding. Navigating these situations while maintaining your dietary commitments requires both practical strategies and psychological preparation [212].

Emily, 33, worked as an event planner, which meant her professional life revolved around food. Tastings with caterers. Client dinners. Networking events where refusing food felt like refusing connection. When she first adopted the protocol, her social anxiety around eating spiked dramatically. 'I feel like I'm being rude,' she told me. 'Like I'm judging everyone else's choices by refusing to participate.'

Emily's discomfort is common. We are social creatures, and food serves purposes far beyond nutrition. But her concern was based on a misunderstanding: protecting your health doesn't mean rejecting connection or judging others. It simply means making different choices while remaining fully present in social situations [213].

The Art of Simple Communication

Most social food pressure dissolves with simple, confident communication. The key is brevity: detailed explanations invite debate, while simple statements typically end conversation [214].

'I'm focusing on protein and vegetables right now' explains your choices without inviting dietary debate.

'I'm cutting out sugar and processed foods for health reasons' satisfies curiosity without requiring you to explain the Toxic Nine or the MILA system.

'My doctor has me on an elimination protocol' suggests medical necessity that most people respect without questioning.

If someone persists in questioning your choices or pressuring you to eat differently, the problem lies with their behavior, not yours. A simple 'This is what works for me' ends most conversations. If it doesn't, feel free to change the subject [215].

Practical Social Strategies

Several strategies reduce social eating pressure:

Eat before arriving. Attending a party or event with a satisfied appetite dramatically reduces temptation. Have a compliant meal before going, so you are not making decisions from a state of hunger [216].

Bring your own contribution. For potlucks and gatherings, bring a dish you can eat, and bring enough for others. Often your contribution will be among the most popular items. Guacamole with vegetables, a beautiful salad with grilled chicken, or grilled vegetable skewers all travel well and appeal broadly [217].

Focus on the people. Remember that the purpose of social gatherings is connection, not consumption. Position yourself away from food tables. Engage in conversations. The food becomes less central when you're focused on relationships.

Hold a drink. Having something in your hand, even sparkling water with lime, reduces the social pressure to be eating or drinking. It gives you something to do during conversations and signals participation without requiring problematic consumption [218].

Accept imperfection strategically. Some situations, grandmother's 90th birthday, your best friend's wedding rehearsal dinner, a once-in-a-lifetime cultural experience, may warrant choosing connection over perfect compliance. This is what your strategic 'cheats' (discussed in the next chapter) are for. The key is making this a conscious choice rather than a default surrender [219].

The Critical Role of Meal Preparation

If there is one factor that predicts success or failure with this protocol, it is preparation. Without planning, you will consistently make poor food choices, not because you lack willpower, but because of how the human brain is wired [220].

When you are hungry and must decide what to eat immediately, your brain defaults to seeking the highest calorie, most immediately available option. This is an evolutionary survival mechanism. Our ancestors who grabbed the quickest calories in times of scarcity survived. But in modern environments with processed food on every corner, this instinct works against you [221].

Research demonstrates that when people wait until they're hungry to decide what to eat, they choose foods 40% higher in calories compared to when they plan meals in advance [222]. If you wait until 6 PM and you're hungry with nothing prepared, you will order pizza. This isn't weakness. This is neuroscience.

The Meal Prep System

Meal preparation means dedicating specific time, typically two to three hours once or twice weekly, to preparing foods in advance. This investment eliminates hours of decision-making and prevents the inevitable poor choices that come from facing hunger without a plan [223].

Proteins: Cook several days' worth at once. Grill or bake six to eight chicken breasts. Prepare a large batch of ground turkey. Hard-boil a dozen eggs. Cook a large piece of salmon to portion throughout the week. Store in glass containers in the refrigerator [224].

Carbohydrates: Cook in bulk and store. A large pot of brown rice refrigerates well for five days. Make a batch of quinoa. Bake four to six sweet potatoes at once. Prepare a slow cooker of beans.

Vegetables: Wash, chop, and store. Pre-cut salad ingredients for quick assembly. Chop vegetables for stir-fries or roasting. Steam broccoli and other vegetables, ready to reheat.

Portioned snacks: Pre-measure nut portions in individual bags to prevent mindless overeating. Wash and prepare fruit. Having grab-and-go options eliminates decision fatigue [223].

Creating Sustainable Systems

Beyond basic meal prep, sustainable success requires systems that make compliance the default rather than a constant effort [225].

Schedule your prep time. Put meal preparation in your calendar as a non-negotiable appointment. Sunday afternoon works for many people, but choose whatever time fits your schedule. Treat it like any other important meeting.

Plan your meals before shopping. Know what you are making before you enter the grocery store. This prevents both forgetting essential items and impulsively buying foods that don't serve your goals [135].

Keep your kitchen stocked. Maintain a list of staples that should always be in your home: olive oil, eggs, frozen vegetables, nuts, whatever proteins you eat regularly. When items run low, they go immediately on the shopping list.

Create default meals. Have three to five simple meals you can make with minimal thought. When you are tired and decision-making feels impossible, these defaults save you. Grilled chicken, steamed broccoli, and brown rice. Salmon with roasted vegetables. Eggs scrambled with whatever vegetables are available. These simple combinations require no recipes and produce reliable results [226].

Use technology. Grocery pick-up and delivery services eliminate the temptation-filled store experience. Meal planning apps can automate the thinking. Set phone reminders for prep time and shopping days.

Optimizing Your Food Environment

Your environment shapes your choices more than your willpower. This is not a character flaw; it is human psychology. The foods visible and easily accessible are the foods you'll eat most often, regardless of your intentions [227].

Remove problematic foods. You cannot eat what isn't there. If ice cream is in your freezer, you'll eventually eat it during a moment of weakness. If it's not there, that moment passes without damage. This isn't about deprivation; it is about removing the need for constant willpower [228].

Make compliant foods visible. Put the fruit bowl on the counter. Store pre-cut vegetables at eye level in the refrigerator. Place nuts in clear containers where you will see them. Visibility drives consumption.

Create convenience. The easier something is to eat, the more you'll eat it. Pre-washed grapes get eaten; grapes still on the stem requiring washing get ignored. Pre-cut vegetables get grabbed; whole vegetables requiring preparation stay unused until they spoil [229].

Reorganize your kitchen. Put cooking oils, spices, and healthy staples where they are easily accessible. Relegate any remaining non-compliant items (if you're living with family members who eat differently) to inconvenient locations. This small friction reduces their use.

When Family Members Eat Differently

One of the most challenging situations patients face is maintaining their dietary commitments when family members aren't following the same protocol. Spouses who want their comfort foods, children who resist anything 'healthy,' extended family who view dietary restrictions as personal rejection, all create genuine obstacles [230].

Helpful Strategies

Cook compliant meals with optional add-ons. Prepare grilled chicken, vegetables, and rice as the base meal. Family members who want bread, cheese, or sauces can add them to their plates. You eat the base meal; others customize theirs [231].

Focus on what you are adding, not removing. Especially with children, emphasize the delicious foods you're eating rather than what's 'forbidden.' Make vegetables appealing through preparation. Let them see you enjoying your food, not suffering through it.

Lead by example. As family members observe your improved energy, weight loss, and reduced symptoms, curiosity often develops. Many patients report that family members gradually adopt aspects of the protocol after seeing results, not because they were convinced through argument [232].

Create compliant versions of family favorites. Tacos become taco salads. Pizza becomes pizza-topped chicken. Pasta dishes become the sauce over vegetables or compliant grains. Creativity maintains family meal togetherness while respecting your needs.

Maintain your boundaries kindly. You are not obligated to eat inflammatory foods to make others comfortable. But you can decline without lecture, refuse without judgment, and protect your health while maintaining loving relationships [233].

When Time Is the Enemy

'I don't have time to cook' ranks among the most common objections to this protocol. Modern life is genuinely busy, and the pressure of competing demands makes food preparation feel like an unaffordable luxury [234].

But consider this reframing: You don't have time not to eat well. The hours lost to brain fog, the days spent sick, the years taken off your life by chronic disease, these costs dwarf the time spent on meal preparation. An hour spent cooking is an hour invested in having more functional hours tomorrow [235].

Practical strategies for time-constrained eating

Simple meals do not require extensive preparation. Grilled chicken, steamed vegetables, and a baked sweet potato take about 30 minutes including prep. Scrambled eggs with vegetables take less than 10 minutes. You're not preparing gourmet cuisine; you are assembling fuel.

Slow cookers allow hands-off cooking. Put ingredients in before work. Dinner is ready when you return. No monitoring required, no standing over a stove.

Sheet pan meals minimize cleanup. Protein and vegetables on a single pan, into the oven, done. One dish to wash.

Batch cooking maximizes efficiency. The time to grill one chicken breast versus six is nearly identical. Cook once, eat several times [236].

Accept help. Pre-cut vegetables, rotisserie chickens (if cooked with acceptable oils), and other convenience items that do not contain inflammatory ingredients save time without sacrificing quality.

Karen's Transformation

Remember Karen, the pharmaceutical sales rep whose traveling lifestyle seemed to make compliance impossible? Her transformation didn't require changing careers. It required changing strategy.

We developed a comprehensive travel protocol. She invested in a quality cooler that fits her carry-on. She researched restaurants near her regular destinations. She identified the grocery stores closest to her most-visited hotels. She developed scripts for ordering at client dinners that sounded normal rather than restrictive.

Most importantly, she stopped viewing travel as an exception to her protocol and started viewing it as simply requiring different strategies within the same protocol. The principles remained constant; only the execution adapted [237].

Within three months, Karen's energy stabilized despite her demanding schedule. Within six months, she had lost 28 pounds. Her fasting blood sugar returned to normal range. Her inflammatory markers dropped dramatically. Her joint pain, which she had assumed was permanent, largely resolved.

'I actually look forward to trips now,' she told me recently. 'I used to dread them because I knew I'd feel terrible afterward. Now I have systems that work. I eat better on the road than most people eat at home. My clients have started asking me about my approach, they see the difference.'

The same transformation is available to anyone willing to apply strategy rather than relying on willpower alone. The real world does not have to defeat your health goals. It simply requires planning, preparation, and the confidence that comes from knowing exactly what to do in any situation [238].

Real-world navigation provides strategies for daily compliance, but what happens when you choose to temporarily step outside the protocol? The reality is that life includes celebrations, cultural experiences, and moments where strict adherence may not serve you.

The next chapter explores the strategic approach to 'cheating,' revealing why how you cheat matters as much as how often, why the biochemistry of the post-cheat period creates unique challenges, and how to contain occasional indulgences to single meals rather than letting them spiral into weeks of abandoned progress.

Understanding this strategic flexibility transforms the protocol from a rigid prison into a sustainable lifestyle.

Key Takeaways

Real-world eating success depends on strategy and preparation rather than willpower because the modern food environment is specifically designed to make inflammatory foods the default choice.

Restaurant dining becomes manageable through simple scripts requesting olive oil preparation and avoiding hidden seed oils in dressings and sauces.

Travel requires pre-planning: packed coolers, researched destinations, and acceptance that imperfect compliance beats complete abandonment.

Social situations need brief, confident responses that protect your choices without inviting debate.

Meal preparation transforms compliance from daily struggle into automatic behavior, eliminating the decision fatigue that leads to poor choices.

The goal is not perfection in impossible circumstances but sustainable progress through practical systems that work in the chaos of actual life.

CHAPTER 8

The Strategic Approach to Cheating

Barbara sat across from me with the unmistakable expression of someone confessing a crime. At 46, this human resources director had been following the protocol with remarkable discipline for four months, experiencing dramatic improvements in her energy, joint pain, and the chronic migraines that had plagued her for years. Then came her daughter's wedding weekend.

'I knew I was going to cheat,' she said. 'I'd planned for it. My daughter's rehearsal dinner, the wedding reception, the brunch the next day. I told myself three meals wouldn't destroy everything I'd built. But here's what I didn't expect.' She paused, collecting herself. 'The wedding was two weeks ago. I haven't been able to get back on track since. Every day I tell myself tomorrow will be different, and every day I find myself eating things I know are destroying my health. It's like something broke inside me.'

Barbara's experience is heartbreakingly common. What she described isn't weakness or lack of willpower. It is biochemistry. The neurological and hormonal cascade triggered by consuming inflammatory foods, particularly sugar, creates a predictable pattern of cravings that can take days or even weeks to resolve. Understanding this biology is essential to developing a strategic approach to the inevitable moments when you choose to step outside the protocol [32].

Because here's the truth that no diet book wants to tell you: you will cheat. Life includes celebrations, traditions, and moments where food carries meaning beyond nutrition. The question isn't whether you'll ever eat outside the protocol. The question is whether those moments will derail months of progress or remain contained exceptions that do not compromise your long-term health [219].

The Reality of Dietary Deviation

Most dietary approaches take one of two extreme positions on 'cheating.' Either they demand perfect compliance, treating any deviation as failure, or they build in regular 'cheat days' that become license for weekly sabotage. Neither approach serves your long-term health [239].

The perfection approach fails because it is unsustainable. Life contains weddings, holidays, travel, and cultural traditions where food plays a central role. Demanding absolute compliance creates two problems: it makes people feel like failures when they inevitably deviate, and it often triggers the 'all or nothing' thinking that turns a single meal into months-long abandonment.

The regular cheat day approach fails because it never allows your body to fully heal and maintains the neurological pathways that drive cravings. Weekly cheat days mean you are perpetually in a cycle of inflammation, recovery, and re-inflammation, never achieving the metabolic stability that comes from sustained compliance [223].

The strategic approach occupies the middle ground: acknowledge that some deviation is inevitable, plan for it thoughtfully, understand the biochemical consequences, and develop strategies to contain those consequences. This isn't permission to cheat regularly. It is recognition that rigid perfection often produces worse outcomes than strategic flexibility [240].

The Six Times Per Year Guideline

For patients following this protocol, the recommended maximum for planned dietary deviations is six times per year. This isn't an arbitrary number. It's based on understanding how the body responds to inflammatory exposure and how long recovery takes [220].

Six occasions spread across a year means roughly one every two months. This allows sufficient time between exposures for inflammatory markers to return to baseline, for the gut microbiome to re-establish healthy populations, and for the neurological cravings triggered by sugar and processed foods to fully subside.

More importantly, six occasions force thoughtful selection. When you know you have limited 'passes,' you choose more carefully. Your child's birthday might make the list. A random Tuesday craving probably won't. This selectivity itself becomes protective, making deviation feel like a conscious choice rather than an impulsive surrender [207].

Some patients ask whether they can 'bank' unused occasions, skipping cheats for several months and then indulging more frequently. The answer is no. The biology does not work that way. What matters is not the total number of deviations but the recovery time between them. Two deviations in the same week caused more damage than six spread throughout the year [222].

What Counts as a Cheat

A strategic cheat is a single meal, not a day, not a weekend, not 'until the holidays are over.' This distinction is crucial. The difference between consuming inflammatory foods at one meal versus multiple meals is enormous in terms of recovery time and craving intensity [218].

When you choose to deviate, eat what you want at that meal, without guilt or restriction. Have the wedding cake. Enjoy your grandmother's traditional holiday dish. Participate fully in the celebration. But when that meal ends, the cheat ends. The next meal returns to full protocol compliance.

This requires planning. If your cheat is dinner at a wedding, ensure your breakfast and lunch that day are fully compliant. Have compliant food ready for the next morning so you are not making decisions while cravings are active. Structure removes the need for willpower during vulnerable moments [211].

The Biochemistry of Cheating

Understanding what happens in your body when you consume inflammatory foods, particularly sugar, explains why the post-cheat period is so difficult and why containment matters so much.

The Dopamine Response

Sugar activates the brain's reward circuitry through dopamine release, the same neurotransmitter involved in addiction to drugs and alcohol. Research using brain imaging has demonstrated that sugar consumption produces effects in the nucleus accumbens, the brain's pleasure center, remarkably similar to cocaine [241].

When you've been avoiding sugar for an extended period, dopamine receptor sensitivity increases. This means when you do consume sugar, the pleasure response is amplified. That wedding cake doesn't just taste good. It triggers a neurological fireworks show that your brain remembers vividly [242].

The problem is what follows. After the dopamine surge comes a crash, and your brain, having experienced that intense pleasure, wants more. Cravings intensify. Foods that seemed satisfying before the cheat now feel bland and unfulfilling. Your brain is quite literally seeking another hit of the substance that produced such reward [243].

The Insulin Cascade

Sugar consumption triggers rapid insulin release to manage the glucose flooding your bloodstream. In someone who has been eating low-sugar whole foods, this insulin response can be dramatic, overcompensating and driving blood sugar lower than optimal. This reactive hypoglycemia creates its own cascade of problems [244].

Low blood sugar signals the brain that you are starving. Hunger intensifies. Energy crashes. Mental fog descends. And the fastest way your brain knows to resolve this emergency is more sugar, creating a cycle where the 'cure' for post-sugar symptoms is more sugar [245].

This cycle can persist for days. Each sugar consumption triggers another insulin spike and crash, perpetuating hunger and cravings that feel uncontrollable. Only by breaking the cycle, by refusing to feed the cravings despite their intensity, can blood sugar stability return.

Ghrelin and Leptin Disruption

Ghrelin, the hunger hormone, and leptin, the satiety hormone, become dysregulated following sugar consumption. Studies demonstrate that high-sugar meals increase subsequent ghrelin secretion while blunting leptin's satiety signals [246]. The result is increased hunger combined with decreased satisfaction from eating, a particularly cruel combination.

This hormonal disruption explains why the day after a cheat, despite eating the same portions that previously felt satisfying, you feel hungrier. Your hormones are literally telling your brain that you haven't eaten enough, even when you have. The signals normalize over several days, but only if you don't keep feeding the disruption [247].

The Inflammatory Response

Beyond the neurological effects, inflammatory foods trigger genuine inflammatory cascades. Seed oils oxidize into aldehydes that damage cell membranes. Gluten increases intestinal permeability in susceptible individuals. Sugar feeds inflammatory bacteria in the gut while starving beneficial species [197].

This inflammation can manifest joint pain returning after months of relief, headaches resuming after a pain-free period, skin conditions flaring, and the general malaise and fatigue that characterized life before the protocol. These symptoms serve as powerful reminders of why the protocol matters, but they're uncomfortable to experience [248].

The inflammatory response also affects mood and cognition. The gut-brain axis means that gut inflammation directly impacts neurotransmitter production and brain function.

Many patients report that the depression and anxiety they thought had resolved returns temporarily after inflammatory food exposure [249].

Understanding the Post-Cheat Period

Frank, 52, managed operations for a manufacturing company. He had been following the protocol for five months with excellent results: 35 pounds lost, blood pressure normalized, and the joint pain that had limited his golf game largely resolved. Then came his company's annual recognition dinner, a black-tie event where he felt obligated to participate fully in the five-course meal and wine pairings.

'I expected to feel bad the next day,' he told me at his follow-up appointment. 'What I didn't expect was how bad, and for how long. The cravings were intense. I felt like I was starting over from day one. My joints hurt again. I was exhausted. And the voice in my head kept saying 'you've already blown it, might as well enjoy the week.'

Frank's experience illustrates why understanding the post-cheat period is so crucial. What he interpreted as 'blowing it' was actually predictable biochemistry. The symptoms were not signs that the protocol had stopped working. They were normal physiological responses to inflammatory exposure. And the voice urging continued indulgence was not rational evaluation. It was dopamine-deprived brain circuitry seeking more stimulation [226].

The Recovery Timeline

After a single-meal cheat, most patients experience the following approximate timeline:

Hours 1–12: Blood sugar fluctuations, possible digestive discomfort, initial inflammation beginning [236].

Hours 12–24: Peak craving intensity as dopamine levels crash and blood sugar seeks stability. This is the most dangerous period for additional cheating. Energy often crashes. Previous symptoms may return (joint pain, headaches, brain fog).

Days 2–3: Cravings remain elevated but begin to diminish. Inflammatory symptoms may peak then begin resolving. Sleep may be disrupted.

Days 4–7: Return to baseline for most people. Cravings subside to manageable levels. Energy stabilizes. Inflammatory symptoms resolve [250].

This timeline extends significantly with multiple-meal or multiple-day cheating. What takes five to seven days to recover from after one meal might take two to three weeks after a weekend of indulgence. This is why containment matters so profoundly. The first cheat triggers biochemistry; additional cheating exponentially extends recovery [251].

The Holiday Trap

No period presents greater danger to dietary progress than the holiday season. What starts as 'just Thanksgiving dinner' can easily become six weeks of continuous inflammatory exposure. Understanding this trap is essential to navigating it successfully [252].

The Holiday Cascade

The pattern is predictable. Thanksgiving dinner leads to Thanksgiving leftovers extending through the weekend. 'It's almost December anyway' provides rationalization for continued deviation. Office holiday parties begin. Christmas cookies appear. Christmas dinner arrives, followed by more leftovers. New Year's Eve celebrations involve food and alcohol. 'I'll start fresh January 2nd' becomes the mantra [253].

This six-week cascade can undo months of progress and reset inflammatory markers to pre-protocol levels. The patient who entered November with normalized blood sugar, reduced inflammation, and stable energy may enter January having regained lost weight, returned to pre-diabetic glucose levels, and experiencing all their previous symptoms [254].

Biochemistry makes the cascade self-perpetuating. Each exposure triggers cravings that make the next exposure more likely. The dopamine system, stimulated repeatedly, demands continued stimulation. What felt like a choice on Thanksgiving becomes compulsion by Christmas [255].

Breaking the Holiday Trap

If you choose to use two of your annual cheats on Thanksgiving and Christmas, make them exactly that: two meals, not six weeks. This requires advance planning and firm commitment [256].

Define your boundaries before the season begins. Decide in advance which meals constitute your cheats. Thanksgiving dinner? Christmas dinner? Some other celebration that matters more to you? Write it down. Commitment in advance is far easier than decision-making in the moment.

Eliminate leftovers. Send remaining food home with guests. Give it away. Dispose of it. Having Thanksgiving leftovers in your refrigerator on Friday morning is setting yourself up for failure. The cheat was the meal; the leftovers are continued exposure [193].

Stock your kitchen with compliant foods. Before the holiday, ensure you have everything needed for compliant meals the following days. Don't let an empty refrigerator provide excuse for continued deviation.

Navigate the in-between events strategically. Office parties, neighbor gatherings, and casual celebrations don't need to be cheats. Eat before attending. Bring a compliant dish to share. Focus on socializing rather than eating. Reserve your actual cheats for the meals that matter most [215].

Recognize rationalization. When you hear yourself thinking 'it's already ruined' or 'I'll start over in January,' recognize this as the addicted brain seeking permission for continued indulgence. Challenge it directly: the protocol isn't ruined, you're in the predictable post-cheat period, and continuing to cheat will only extend the recovery.

Strategies for Successful Containment

Lisa, 39, worked as an attorney specializing in corporate law. Her schedule was demanding, her stress levels were high, and her relationship with food had always been complicated. When she started the protocol, we discussed the inevitability of occasional deviation and developed a comprehensive strategy for containment.

'I'm a planner by nature,' she explained. 'If I know what to expect and have a system, I can manage almost anything. It's the unexpected that derails me.'

Lisa's insight applies broadly. Successful containment isn't about summoning willpower in the moment of craving. It's about building systems in advance that reduce the need for willpower [257].

Pre-Cheat Preparation

Plan your recovery meals. Before the cheat occurs, know exactly what you'll eat for the next three meals. Have these foods in your home prepared if possible. When cravings hit, you're not making decisions; you're executing a plan [258].

Eat compliant meals before the cheat meal. Don't 'save calories' for the event by skipping meals. Arriving hungry intensifies the indulgence and extends the biochemical consequences. A solid protein-based breakfast and lunch before a dinner cheat reduces both consumption and impact.

Hydrate thoroughly. Proper hydration before, during, and after helps the body process inflammatory foods and reduces some of the negative effects [259].

Post-Cheat Protocol

Return immediately to protocol. The next meal after your cheat should be fully compliant. Not tomorrow. Not Monday. The very next meal. Every additional non-compliant meal extends recovery exponentially [221].

Expect and accept discomfort. You will feel cravings. You may experience returning symptoms. Your energy might crash. Accept this as the predictable cost of the cheat rather than evidence that something is wrong.

Increase protein and fat at subsequent meals. Higher protein and fat content promotes satiety and helps stabilize blood sugar, reducing the intensity of cravings. Don't try to 'compensate' by eating less; focus on eating compliant foods until satisfied [216].

Move your body. Exercise helps regulate blood sugar, improves mood through natural endorphin release, and provides a healthy alternative to feeding cravings. Even a 20-minute walk can help break the craving cycle [260].

Stay occupied. Idle time with active cravings is dangerous. Plan activities, work on projects, engage socially. Distraction isn't avoidance; it's strategic management of a temporary biochemical state.

The Taste Bud Transformation and Its Reversal

One aspect of cheating that catches patients off guard is how it temporarily reverses the taste transformation they've experienced on the protocol.

After about 30 days of reduced sugar intake, taste perception shifts dramatically. Fruits taste sweeter. Vegetables develop nuanced flavors previously unnoticed. Foods that once seemed bland become satisfying. This isn't imagination; it's biology. Taste buds regenerate approximately every 10 to 14 days, and new taste buds developed in a low-sugar environment are more sensitive to sweetness [261].

A cheat meal, especially one heavy in sugar, partially reverses this adaptation. Suddenly, the foods that had become satisfying seemed bland again. Fruit doesn't seem sweet enough. Vegetables taste boring. The brain has been reminded of intense sweetness and recalibrated accordingly [261].

This recalibration is temporary, but it contributes to the difficulty of the post-cheat period. Not only are you fighting hormonal cravings, but your actual perception of food has shifted to make compliant options less appealing. Understanding this helps patients push through without assuming they've permanently lost their appreciation for whole foods [262].

The taste transformation returns with continued compliance. Within one to two weeks, sensitivity to natural sweetness restores. Whole food becomes satisfying again. But this window of reduced enjoyment is another reason why containment matters so much. Extended cheating extends the period of diminished appreciation for healthy food [263].

When Cheating Signals Something Deeper

Sometimes the urge to cheat represents more than simple craving or social pressure. Repeated inability to maintain the protocol despite understanding its importance may signal underlying issues that deserve attention [264].

Emotional eating patterns: If cheating consistently follows emotional stress, relationship conflicts, or difficult life events, the food isn't really about food. It's about emotional regulation. Addressing the underlying emotional needs through therapy, stress management, or other support may be more effective than dietary strategies alone [265].

Insufficient nutrition: Persistent cravings sometimes indicate that nutritional needs aren't being met. Inadequate protein, insufficient calories for activity level, or micronutrient deficiencies can all drive cravings that willpower alone can't overcome. Reviewing your actual intake with attention to these factors may reveal fixable problems.

Perfectionism and restriction: Paradoxically, being too strict can trigger more frequent cheating. When the protocol feels like punishment rather than nourishment, rebellion is predictable. If you find yourself swinging between rigid control and complete abandonment, a more moderate approach may produce better long-term results [266].

Unaddressed food addiction: For some individuals, the relationship with certain foods, particularly sugar, meets criteria for addiction. The inability to moderate, the continued use despite negative consequences, and the loss of control despite genuine desire to stop are hallmarks of addictive patterns. These situations may require more structured support than self-management alone can provide [267].

Barbara's Recovery

Remember Barbara from the beginning of this chapter? She was trapped in a two-week spiral following her daughter's wedding. Her recovery began with understanding that what she was experiencing wasn't failure. It was biochemistry.

'When you explained the dopamine and insulin cycles, something clicked,' she told me later. 'I wasn't weak. I was in a predictable chemical state. That reframe changed everything. Instead of beating myself up, which only made me want more comfort food, I could treat it as a temporary situation to manage.'

We developed a structured return protocol. She committed to three days of strict compliance, knowing the cravings would be intense. She prepared all her meals in advance. She scheduled walks during the times she typically felt most vulnerable. She told her husband what she was doing and asked for his support.

The first day was difficult. The second day was harder. But by day three, the cravings began to subside. By the end of the week, she felt back in control. Within two weeks, her energy had returned, her symptoms had resolved, and her taste preferences had recalibrated [237].

'I don't regret enjoying my daughter's wedding,' Barbara said. 'That was worth it. What I regret is the two weeks of suffering that followed because I didn't understand what was happening or have a plan for recovery. If I'd contained it to those three meals, I'd have been back on track within a week.'

Barbara's insight captures the essence of strategic cheating. The goal isn't to never deviate. It's to deviate consciously, contain the deviation to a single meal, understand the biochemical consequences, and have systems in place for rapid return to the protocol [238].

Strategic cheating addresses the planned deviations you choose to make. But what about the foods that trigger reactions even when they're technically 'allowed' on the protocol? Some individuals react to foods outside the Toxic Nine with symptoms just as severe as those caused by the inflammatory foods we've discussed. The next chapter explores food sensitivity testing, the critical difference between IgE allergies and IgG sensitivities, and how to identify your personal trigger foods without falling into the trap of unnecessary elimination that leaves you eating nothing at all. Understanding your unique reactive patterns allows for a truly personalized approach to nutrition.

Key Takeaways

Strategic cheating acknowledges that some dietary deviation is inevitable and plans for it thoughtfully rather than demanding impossible perfection or permitting regular sabotage.

The six times per year guideline allows meaningful participation in celebrations while maintaining healing progress.

Each cheat should be a single meal, not a day or weekend, with immediate return to protocol compliance.

The post-cheat period involves predictable biochemistry, including dopamine crashes, insulin fluctuations, and disrupted hunger hormones, which creates intense cravings lasting four to seven days.

The holiday season presents particular danger, as a cascade from Thanksgiving through New Year's can undo months of progress.

Understanding that post-cheat symptoms represent temporary biochemistry rather than personal failure enables patients to weather the discomfort without spiraling into extended abandonment of the protocol.

CHAPTER 9

Food Sensitivity Testing

Andrea arrived at my office with a list. As a 41-year-old nonprofit director, she approached everything with meticulous organization, and her health journey was no exception. The list contained 47 foods she had eliminated from her diet over the past three years, each one suspected of causing persistent symptoms: migraines, bloating, joint pain, and the chronic fatigue that made her demanding job increasingly difficult.

'I've done everything right,' she said, sliding the list across my desk. 'I eliminated gluten five years ago after reading about it online. Then dairy when that didn't completely fix things. Then eggs after a naturopath suggested them. Then nightshades after a friend said they were inflammatory. Then histamines after an article I read. Then FODMAPs after a gastroenterologist recommended them.' She paused, frustration evident in her voice. 'I'm basically eating chicken, rice, and a handful of vegetables. I'm losing weight, I don't need to lose. I'm exhausted. And I still have symptoms.'

Andrea's story represents a growing problem in the health-conscious community: elimination without evidence. In an effort to identify trigger foods, she had progressively restricted her diet based on symptoms that might or might not have been connected to specific foods, advice from well-meaning but uninformed sources, and assumptions that never underwent actual testing [268].

The result was not better health. It was malnutrition, social isolation around food, and symptoms that persisted despite her sacrifices. What Andrea needed was not more elimination. She needed strategic testing to identify her actual reactive foods, not the foods she assumed were problems [269].

The Problem with Assumed Food Sensitivities

When patients experience symptoms, they suspect are food-related, the natural impulse is to identify the culprit and eliminate it. This instinct is sound. The problem is how that identification typically happens: through assumption, coincidence, or well-meaning but unreliable advice [270].

'I had a headache after eating tomatoes, so I must be sensitive to tomatoes.' Perhaps. Or perhaps the headache came from dehydration, stress, poor sleep, the wine with dinner, the aged cheese in the sauce, or any dozens of other factors. Without controlled testing, a single correlation becomes assumed causation, and another food disappears from the diet unnecessarily [271].

The consequences of unnecessary elimination extend beyond inconvenience. Nutritional deficiencies develop as food variety shrinks. Social eating becomes fraught with anxiety. The psychological burden of managing an increasingly restricted diet creates its own stress, which ironically can worsen symptoms. And perhaps most problematically, the actual trigger foods may remain in the diet while innocent foods take the blame [270].

Understanding Food Reactions: Types and Mechanisms

Not all negative food reactions are created equal. Understanding the different types of reactions helps explain why testing matters and why self-diagnosis so often fails.

IgE Allergies: The Immediate Response

True food allergies involve Immunoglobulin E (IgE) antibodies and produce immediate, often severe reactions. When someone with a peanut allergy consumes peanuts, their immune system recognizes peanut proteins as dangerous invaders and triggers an immediate cascade of histamine release and inflammatory responses [272].

Symptoms of IgE reactions typically appear within minutes to two hours and can include hives, swelling, difficulty breathing, gastrointestinal distress, and in severe cases, anaphylaxis. These reactions are usually unmistakable. You don't wonder whether you're having an allergic reaction; you know [273].

IgE allergies are relatively easy to diagnose through skin prick tests or blood tests measuring IgE antibodies to specific foods. They are also relatively rare, affecting approximately 2-4% of adults [274].

IgG Sensitivities: The Delayed Response

Food sensitivities, in contrast to allergies, involve Immunoglobulin G (IgG) antibodies and produce delayed reactions that can occur anywhere from several hours to several days after consumption. This delay makes self-identification extremely difficult. How do you connect Tuesday's migraine to Sunday's meal [275]?

IgG reactions tend to produce more diffuse, systemic symptoms: headaches, joint pain, brain fog, fatigue, skin issues, digestive complaints, and mood disturbances. These symptoms overlap with countless other conditions, further complicating identification [276].

Other Reaction Types

Enzyme deficiencies like lactose intolerance occur when the body lacks enzymes to properly digest certain compounds. These deficiencies produce symptoms with predictable foods [277].

Histamine intolerance involves difficulty processing histamine found naturally in certain foods or produced by gut bacteria [278].

FODMAP sensitivity relates to fermentable carbohydrates that cause digestive symptoms in susceptible individuals [279].

The Value of Proper Testing

Kenneth, 59, worked as a contractor. His hands, essential to his livelihood, had become increasingly painful and swollen over the past several years. His doctor diagnosed early rheumatoid arthritis and started him on medications. A friend suggested his diet might be contributing and recommended eliminating gluten.

Kenneth dutifully removed all gluten from his diet. When improvement did not come, he eliminated dairy. Then nightshades. Then eggs. Each elimination came with hope that faded as symptoms persisted. By the time he came to see me, he had eliminated so many foods that his diet consisted primarily of rice, fish, and a handful of vegetables.

We ran comprehensive food sensitivity testing. The results surprised us both. Kenneth showed no significant reaction to gluten, dairy, or night shades. But he showed strong IgG reactions to almonds and chicken, foods he was eating almost daily [280].

We reintroduced nightshades and other foods on the R.E.S.T.O.R.E MILA Protocol while eliminating almonds and chicken. Within three weeks, his hand swelling decreased noticeably. Within two months, his pain had reduced enough that his rheumatologist reduced his medication. The foods he had sacrificed for years were never the problem.

The Two-Part Testing Approach

Effective food sensitivity identification requires a two-part approach: laboratory testing to identify likely culprits, followed by systematic elimination and reintroduction to confirm clinical significance [281].

Part One: Laboratory Testing

IgG food sensitivity panels measure antibody levels to various foods, typically testing 96 to 200+ items. When the immune system repeatedly encounters a food, it perceives it as problematic, it produces antibodies that can be measured in blood [282].

It is important to understand what these tests do and do not tell you. A positive IgG result indicates that your immune system has mounted a response to that food. It doesn't definitively prove that food causes your symptoms [283].

Part Two: Elimination and Reintroduction

Once testing identifies foods with elevated antibody levels, the next step is systematic elimination followed by careful reintroduction. This clinical confirmation separates foods that actually cause symptoms from those that produce antibodies without clinical significance [284].

The elimination phase removes all reactive foods for a period of three to four weeks, enough time for antibody levels to decrease and symptoms to potentially resolve [285].

There are three categories of food that typically take up to 6 months before reintroduction — if at all: dairy, gluten, and eggs. These often cause mimicry, meaning that once we have sensitivities to these foods our bodies often attack ourselves. Reintroduction of these three often causes a quick exacerbation of symptoms.

The reintroduction phase adds food back one at a time, with at least three days between reintroductions to allow delayed reactions to manifest [284].

Common Testing Pitfalls

Testing Foods You Don't Eat: IgG antibodies require exposure to develop. If you have not eaten a food in several months, your antibody levels may have declined regardless of whether you're actually sensitive [286].

Over-Interpreting Results: Not every elevated antibody represents a clinically significant sensitivity. Mild elevations may simply reflect regular exposure rather than pathological response.

Incomplete Elimination: Many foods hide in unexpected places. Dairy appears as casein, whey, and lactose in countless products.

Rushing Reintroduction: The 72-hour window between reintroductions exists because IgG reactions can be delayed.

The Danger of Over-Elimination

Samantha, 35, taught elementary school and had always been conscientious about her health. When she developed chronic bloating and fatigue, she began eliminating foods she read might be problematic. By the time she came to see me, she had been on an increasingly restrictive diet for six years.

Her current diet included only about fifteen foods. She was significantly underweight. Her hair had thinned noticeably. Lab work revealed multiple nutritional deficiencies: iron, B12, vitamin D, zinc, and omega-3 fatty acids.

Samantha had fallen into a trap that catches many well-intentioned patients. Her elimination had become so severe that her digestive system had lost the capacity to handle normal foods. The 'reactions' she experienced when trying to reintroduce foods were often not sensitivities at all but the predictable response of a gut unaccustomed to variety [287].

The Gut Connection

Food sensitivities do not develop in isolation. They often reflect underlying gut dysfunction, particularly increased intestinal permeability, sometimes called 'leaky gut.' When the gut barrier becomes compromised, food particles that should remain in the digestive tract enter the bloodstream, triggering immune responses [286].

This connection has important implications. First, addressing gut health often reduces food sensitivities over time. Foods that were reactive during active gut dysfunction may become tolerable once the gut heals [287].

The R.E.S.T.O.R.E. protocol addresses this comprehensively. By supporting gut healing through the elimination of the Toxic Nine and the restoration of gut integrity, many patients find their food sensitivity list shrinks naturally over time [288].

Andrea's Restoration

Remember Andrea, who arrived with her list of 47 eliminated foods? Her testing revealed only four significant sensitivities: eggs, almonds, oats, and yeast. Of the 47 foods she had eliminated, 43 showed no significant reaction.

Following the two-part approach, Andrea eliminated her four reactive foods while carefully reintroducing the others. Nightshades, which she had avoided for two years, produced no symptoms. Even meats, after careful reintroduction, caused no issues.

She gained needed weight. Her energy improved as her nutrition normalized. Her social life around food rekindled. And her actual trigger foods, now identified and eliminated, no longer caused the symptoms that had driven her restrictive spiral.

Accessing Food Sensitivity Testing

Food sensitivity testing is available through various sources. The Dynamic Intake at restoremila.com can help identify whether food sensitivity testing is indicated for your situation and provide guidance on appropriate testing options [289].

Identifying reactive foods addresses what you eat, but equally important is the quality of what you consume.

The next chapter explores why source matters profoundly for animal products: how conventional farming practices create inflammatory, nutritionally depleted foods; why the health of the animal directly impacts the health of the human who consumes it; and how choosing pasture-raised, grass-fed, and wild-caught options transforms the same foods from inflammatory to healing.

Understanding the difference between factory-farmed and traditionally raised animal products reveals why spending more at the grocery store often means spending less at the doctor's office.

Key Takeaways

Food sensitivity identification requires testing rather than assumption because delayed IgG reactions can occur hours to days after consumption, making self-identification unreliable.

The two-part approach combines laboratory testing to identify likely reactive foods with systematic elimination and reintroduction to confirm clinical significance.

Not every elevated antibody causes symptoms, and not every symptom comes from suspected foods, so clinical confirmation matters more than test results alone.

Over-elimination based on untested assumptions leads to nutritional deficiencies, compromised gut function, and continued symptoms from actual trigger foods that remain unidentified.

Many sensitivities improve as gut health restores, making permanent elimination unnecessary for foods that were reactive during active dysfunction.

The goal is identifying your genuine trigger foods while preserving the dietary diversity essential for optimal nutrition and quality of life.

CHAPTER 10

Animal Product Quality

Howard had been a police officer for 30 years before retiring at 54. He prided himself on his physical fitness, maintaining the same workout routine he had followed throughout his career. But despite his disciplined exercise habits, his health had deteriorated significantly over the past decade. His cholesterol required medication. His blood pressure had crept up. Joint pain had become a constant companion. And the fatigue that settled over him each afternoon made him feel decades older than his years.

'I eat healthy,' he insisted during our first appointment. 'Chicken breast every day for lunch. Eggs every morning. Fish twice a week. Lots of protein, just like I was taught in the academy. But something's not working.'

When I asked about the source of his protein, Howard looked confused. 'The grocery store. Regular chicken. Regular eggs. What else is there?'

What Howard didn't understand, and what most patients fail to realize, is that the same food can be inflammatory or anti-inflammatory depending entirely on how it was raised. The chicken breast from a concentrated animal feeding operation (CAFO) is a fundamentally different food, at the molecular level, than chicken from a bird raised on pasture. Understanding this difference transforms how you approach protein selection and explains why source matters as much as the food itself.

The CAFO Revolution and Its Consequences

Before the 1950s, virtually all animal products came from animals raised on farms, eating their natural diets, with access to pasture, sunshine, and space to move. The chicken was a chicken; a cow was a cow. Quality varied by farm, but the fundamental nature of the animal and its products remained consistent with thousands of years of human dietary history.

The concentrated animal feeding operation changed everything. Driven by economic pressure to produce more protein faster and cheaper, the CAFO model confines thousands of animals in minimal space, feeds them diets optimized for rapid weight gain rather than health, and uses pharmaceutical intervention to keep animals alive long enough to reach slaughter weight [290].

The scale of this transformation is staggering. Today, over 99% of chickens, 97% of laying hens, 99% of turkeys, 95% of pigs, and 78% of cattle in the United States are raised in CAFOs. The 'farm' of popular imagination, with animals grazing on green pastures, represents a tiny fraction of actual animal agriculture [291].

What CAFO Animals Eat

In nature, chickens are omnivores that eat insects, seeds, grass, and whatever they find while scratching the ground. Cattle are ruminants designed to eat grass, with complex digestive systems that evolved specifically for fermenting fibrous plant material. Pigs forage widely, consuming roots, vegetation, and the occasional protein source.

In CAFOs, these animals eat something entirely different. The primary feed is corn and soybeans, often genetically modified and grown with pesticide applications that leave residues in the grain. This diet is supplemented with various additives: rendered animal parts, growth promoters, and medications [291].

For cattle, corn feeding creates particular problems. The bovine digestive system evolved to process grass, not grain. Corn feeding causes acidosis, a painful condition where the rumen becomes too acidic, damaging the stomach lining and allowing bacteria to enter the bloodstream. To manage this, CAFO cattle receive constant low-dose antibiotics [291].

The Antibiotic Crisis

Approximately 80% of all antibiotics sold in the United States are used in animal agriculture, not for treating sick animals but for promoting growth and preventing the diseases that inevitably arise in crowded, unsanitary conditions [292].

This massive antibiotic use drives the development of antibiotic-resistant bacteria. Animals become reservoirs for resistant strains that can transfer to humans through direct contact, environmental contamination, and consumption. The connection between agricultural antibiotic use and the rise of drug-resistant infections is well established [291].

But beyond the public health implications of antibiotic resistance, the antibiotics themselves end up in the meat you eat. While regulations require withdrawal periods before slaughter, residue remains. You're consuming small amounts of antibiotics with every CAFO animal product, affecting your own gut microbiome [291].

Hormones and Growth Promoters

To accelerate growth and increase profitability, many CAFO operations use hormones and hormone-like compounds. Cattle commonly receive estrogen, progesterone, testosterone, or synthetic equivalents. Dairy cows often receive recombinant bovine growth hormone (rBGH) to increase milk production [87].

These hormones do not disappear when the animal is processed. They concentrate in the fat and end up on your plate. Research links consumption of hormone-treated animal products to early puberty, reproductive abnormalities, and increased cancer risk [291].

The Supporting Case: Janet

Janet, 47, worked as an office manager and had struggled with weight and hormonal issues throughout her adult life. She had been diagnosed with polycystic ovary syndrome in her twenties and had experienced difficulty conceiving. Now, in perimenopause, her symptoms had intensified. Hot flashes, mood swings, and stubborn weight around her midsection made daily life challenging.

'I've already cut out so many things,' she told me. 'No more fast food. No processed foods. I cook at home almost every night. But I'm not seeing the improvement I expected.'

When we reviewed her diet, Janet was eating plenty of protein, chicken, beef, and eggs. But all of it came from conventional sources, the cheapest options at her local grocery store. Her daily exposure to the hormones, antibiotics, and inflammatory fatty acid profiles of CAFO products was significant [293].

Switching to pasture-raised eggs, grass-fed beef, and organic chicken represented a meaningful financial investment. But within two months, Janet's hot flashes had decreased substantially. Her mood stabilized. And the stubborn weight, which had resisted all previous efforts, began to shift. 'I'm eating the same amount of food,' she noted. 'Just better versions of it.'

The Nutritional Difference

The difference between CAFO and pasture-raised animal products extends far beyond what the animals are exposed to. It fundamentally changes the nutritional profile of the food itself [294].

Fatty Acid Composition

The fat composition of animal products directly reflects what the animal ate. Grass-fed beef contains dramatically different fatty acids than grain-fed beef from the same breed of cattle [290].

Grass-fed beef contains two to five times more omega-3 fatty acids than grain-fed beef. It contains significantly higher levels of conjugated linoleic acid (CLA), a fatty acid associated with reduced inflammation and improved body composition. And it has a much healthier omega-6 to omega-3 ratio, typically around 2:1 compared to 20:1 or higher in grain-fed beef [295].

This matters because fatty acids aren't just calories. They are signaling molecules that influence inflammation, hormone production, and cell membrane function throughout your body. Consuming animal products with wildly distorted fatty acid profiles creates inflammation at the cellular level [296].

The same pattern applies to eggs. Pasture-raised eggs from hens that eat insects, grass, and their natural diet contain significantly more omega-3s, more vitamins A, D, and E, and more beta-carotene than eggs from confined hens eating only grain [297].

Vitamin and Mineral Content

Animals raised on pasture, with access to sunshine and diverse vegetation, produce foods with higher vitamin and mineral content. Grass-fed beef contains significantly more vitamin A, vitamin E, and B vitamins than grain-fed beef [295].

Pasture-raised eggs have darker, more orange yolks, reflecting their higher carotenoid content. They contain more vitamin D because the hens spend time in sunlight, and more vitamin E from the diverse vegetation in their diet [298].

Bioaccumulation: You Are What You Eat Ate

Toxins accumulate in fat tissue. When animals eat contaminated feed, pesticide residues, heavy metals, and other toxins concentrate in their fat. This process, called bioaccumulation, means that consuming animal fat from conventionally raised animals delivers concentrated doses of whatever toxins those animals were exposed to [297].

CAFO animals, fed grain grown with pesticides and raised in environments where industrial chemicals are common, accumulate these substances in their fat tissue. When you eat that fat, whether in meat, dairy, or eggs, you are consuming those concentrated toxins [297].

Pasture-raised animals, eating diverse vegetation in cleaner environments, have lower toxic burdens. Their fat is not only nutritionally superior but also less contaminated with industrial chemicals and pesticide residues.

Making the Transition

Prioritizing Your Purchases

Not everyone can afford to transition all animal products to pasture-raised overnight. A strategic approach prioritizes the food that matters most.

Eggs represent perhaps the best value upgrade. Pasture-raised eggs cost more than conventional, but the price difference is modest compared to meat. Given that many people eat eggs daily and given the dramatic nutritional superiority of pasture-raised eggs, this should be the first transition.

Beef and dairy represent the next priority. Fat-soluble toxins, hormones, and the fatty acid composition all make grass-fed beef and organic dairy important upgrades. If budget is limited, prioritize beef over chicken, as conventional beef often contains more hormones [87].

Chicken and pork, while still worth upgrading, typically contain fewer added hormones than beef due to different regulations. Organic or pasture-raised options remain preferable but may be lower priority when budget is constrained.

Finding Quality Sources

Pasture-raised and grass-fed products are increasingly available in mainstream grocery stores. Look for specific certifications: 'Grass-fed' for beef, 'Pasture-raised' for eggs and poultry. Be aware that marketing terms like 'natural' or 'farm fresh' are essentially meaningless [295].

Local farmers markets often provide access to small-scale producers who raise animals traditionally. These products may not carry official certifications but may exceed certified products in quality. Talking directly with farmers about their practices provides information labels can't convey.

Online sources have expanded options for those without local access. Various companies ship grass-fed beef and pasture-raised products directly to consumers, sometimes at competitive prices with grocery store options.

Gregory's Transformation

Gregory, 63, was a retired teacher who had been diagnosed with elevated inflammatory markers during a routine checkup. His doctor was concerned about his cardiovascular risk and recommended medication. Gregory wanted to try dietary changes first.

Beyond eliminating the Toxic Nine, we focused specifically on upgrading his animal product sources. He had been eating conventional meat and eggs almost exclusively. The transition to grass-fed beef, pasture-raised eggs, and wild-caught fish represented a significant dietary shift.

At his six-month follow-up, Gregory's inflammatory markers had dropped significantly. His CRP, a measure of systemic inflammation, had decreased by over 50%. His HDL cholesterol had improved while his LDL had decreased. His doctor was impressed enough to postpone medication discussions.

'I'm eating basically the same foods,' Gregory observed. 'Same amounts, same proteins, same meals. Simply better quality. The price difference was real, but so are my lab results. I can't argue with the numbers.'

Wild-Caught Versus Farm-Raised Fish

The same principles that apply to land animals apply to fish. Wild-caught fish eat their natural diets and live in their natural environments. Farm-raised fish are often crowded in pens, fed unnatural diets, and given antibiotics to prevent disease [142].

Farm-raised salmon, one of the most common farmed fish, typically contains higher levels of pollutants like PCBs and dioxins than wild salmon. The flesh is artificially colored because the natural diet that produces salmon's pink color is absent. And the fatty acid profile, while still containing omega-3s, is less favorable than wild-caught [298].

Wild-caught fish, particularly cold-water species like salmon, sardines, and mackerel, provide omega-3 fatty acids in their natural ratios and forms. These should be prioritized over farm-raised alternatives whenever possible.

The quality of your food sources reveals one pathway to health that traditional cultures have followed for millennia. The next chapter examines the Blue Zones, regions around the world where people routinely live past 100 in good health, and what their dietary patterns reveal about the principles we've discussed. These populations never read nutrition studies or worried about inflammatory markers, yet they naturally avoided the Toxic Nine and consumed high-quality animal products in patterns that modern science is only now validating. Their lived experience provides compelling proof that ancestral eating patterns promote exceptional longevity.

Key Takeaways

Animal product quality matters as much as what animal products you choose because CAFO-raised animals produce nutritionally depleted, inflammatory food regardless of the species.

Conventional animal agriculture relies on unnatural diets, antibiotics, and hormones that fundamentally alter the fatty acid profiles, nutrient content, and toxic burden of meat, dairy, and eggs.

Grass-fed beef contains dramatically more omega-3 fatty acids and conjugated linoleic acid while having healthier omega-6 to omega-3 ratios compared to grain-fed alternatives.

Pasture-raised eggs provide significantly more vitamins, carotenoids, and healthy fats than eggs from confined hens.

Bioaccumulation concentrates toxins in animal fat, making the quality of what animals eat directly relevant to your own toxic exposure.

Strategic prioritization, starting with eggs and grass-fed beef, allows gradual transition to higher-quality sources within budget constraints.

CHAPTER 11

Blue Zones

I had the pleasure of meeting Vincent as he settled into the chair across from me with the ease of a man at peace with his body. At 72, this retired professor of anthropology still climbed the steep hills near his home in southern Italy each week, tended his vegetable garden daily, and walked to the local market most mornings. His posture was straight, his eyes clear, his handshake firm. He had come to see me not because of illness, but because his American-born daughter had become concerned about her own health and wanted her father's perspective included in her treatment plan.

'She tells me I need to explain my diet to you,' Vincent said with a gentle smile. 'But there is nothing to explain. I eat what my grandmother ate. What her grandmother ate. What people in my village have eaten for centuries. It never occurred to anyone that this required an explanation until my daughter started reading American nutrition books.'

Vincent had grown up in a region of Italy that researchers would later identify as a longevity hotspot, an area where the concentration of centenarians far exceeded statistical expectations. He had unknowingly followed dietary patterns that modern science is only now validating, not through study or discipline, but simply by eating the way his culture had always eaten [394].

His story illustrates a profound irony: the populations with the best health outcomes have never heard of elimination diets, macronutrient ratios, or anti-inflammatory protocols. They simply eat real food, the same food their ancestors ate, and live longer, healthier lives than populations with access to modern medicine and nutrition science [395].

What Are the Blue Zones?

The term 'Blue Zones' was coined by researcher Dan Buettner to describe five regions around the world where people live significantly longer than average and experience dramatically lower rates of chronic disease. These regions include Okinawa, Japan; Sardinia, Italy; Nicoya Peninsula, Costa Rica; Ikaria, Greece; and Loma Linda, California [396].

What makes these regions remarkable isn't just that people live longer. It's that they live better. Centenarians in Blue Zones typically remain active and independent into their final years. The extended period of disability and decline that characterizes aging in industrialized societies is largely absent. People don't just add years to their lives; they add life to their years [397].

Researchers studying these populations have identified multiple contributing factors: strong social connections, regular physical activity built into daily life, sense of purpose, stress-reduction practices, and, crucially, distinct dietary patterns. While the specific foods vary by region, the underlying principles remain remarkably consistent.

Natural Avoidance of the Toxic Nine

Perhaps the most striking feature of Blue Zone diets is what they don't contain. These traditional eating patterns naturally exclude most or all of the Toxic Nine, not because of any conscious health decision but because these foods simply were not part of traditional diets.

Sugar

Traditional Blue Zone diets contain minimal added sugar. Sweetness came from fruit, honey used sparingly, or naturally sweet vegetables like sweet potatoes. The average Okinawan centenarian grew up consuming a tiny fraction of the sugar consumed by modern Americans [59].

When researchers measured the sugar intake of traditional Okinawans, they found consumption levels of roughly 5-10 pounds per year, compared to the 150+ pounds consumed by average Americans today. This difference alone represents a massive reduction in inflammatory exposure.

Wheat and Gluten

While some Blue Zones, particularly in the Mediterranean, include bread, the bread bears no resemblance to modern wheat products. Traditional Sardinian bread is made from ancient grain varieties, slowly fermented using traditional sourdough methods that partially break down gluten and phytates [238].

Okinawan and Costa Rican Blue Zones barely consumed wheat at all. Their carbohydrate sources were rice, sweet potatoes, and corn prepared through traditional methods (like nixtamalization) that improve digestibility and nutrient availability.

Processed Corn and Soy

The processed corn derivatives and soy isolates that pervade modern processed foods are entirely absent from Blue Zone diets. While traditional Okinawans consumed fermented soy (miso, tofu, tempeh), the fermentation process transforms the soy into a different nutritional entity. And no Blue Zone population consumed high fructose corn syrup, corn oil, or soy protein isolates because these industrial products didn't exist [62].

Conventional Dairy

Dairy consumption varies across Blue Zones. Some Mediterranean Blue Zones include sheep and goat milk products, typically fermented into cheese or yogurt. These products come from pastured animals eating their natural diets, and the fermentation process alters the protein structure. Okinawan and Costa Rican Blue Zones consume little to no dairy [59].

Notably absent from all Blue Zones is the industrialized, hormone-laden, A1-casein-dominant dairy that characterizes modern consumption. When dairy is present, it's a fundamentally different product than what fills American grocery shelves.

Peanuts and Seed Oils

Blue Zone populations consume no industrial seed oils. Their fats come from olive oil (Mediterranean zones), coconut (Okinawa), or small amounts of animal fat. The omega-6 overload created by modern seed oil consumption is entirely absent from these traditional diets.

Peanuts play no significant role in any Blue Zone diet. Nut consumption, where present, centers on tree nuts like almonds, walnuts, or cashews.

Alcohol (with Exceptions)

Alcohol consumption in Blue Zones is minimal or absent. The notable exception is Sardinia, where moderate red wine consumption (one to two glasses daily, typically with meals) is common. However, this represents the controlled, social consumption of a single, traditionally produced beverage, not the varied and excessive alcohol consumption common in modern societies.

Chemical Additives

Traditional Blue Zone diets contain zero chemical preservatives, artificial colors, artificial flavors, or emulsifiers. Food is fresh, local, seasonal, and unprocessed. The 140+ pounds of food additives consumed annually by average Americans simply don't exist in these dietary patterns [48].

Dorothy's Discovery

Dorothy, 78, had worked as a nurse for over four decades. She had seen countless patients suffer from chronic diseases and had watched medical interventions provide, at best, management rather than cure. As she entered her own senior years, she was determined to approach aging differently.

'I've spent my career watching people get sicker despite doing everything their doctors told them,' she explained. 'I wanted to understand why some people stay healthy into their eighties and nineties while others fall apart in their sixties.'

Dorothy's research led her to Blue Zone literature. What she found confirmed her clinical observations: the populations with the best health outcomes weren't following medical advice. They were simply eating traditional diets that happened to exclude everything modern medicine was trying to treat.

She began adopting Blue Zone principles. At 78, she had more energy than she had at 60. Her joint pain, which she had assumed was inevitable aging, had largely resolved. Her blood pressure, previously requiring medication, had normalized. 'The answer was so simple,' she reflected. 'Eat real food. Move your body. Stay connected to people. It's not complicated, it's just not profitable for anyone to tell you.'

The Okinawan Experiment

Perhaps no population provides more striking evidence of the diet-health connection than the Okinawans, because their story includes a natural experiment that demonstrates what happens when traditional eating patterns are abandoned.

For most of the 20th century, Okinawa had the highest concentration of centenarians in the world. The traditional Okinawan diet centered on sweet potatoes, vegetables, tofu, small amounts of fish, and minimal meat. Sugar consumption was low. Processed foods were essentially nonexistent.

Then came the American military presence following World War II. Fast food restaurants arrived. Processed foods became available. Young Okinawans, particularly those near military bases, adopted Western eating patterns.

The result has been a dramatic decline in Okinawan longevity. While elders who maintained traditional diets continued to exhibit remarkable health spans, younger generations consuming Western diets began developing Western diseases at Western rates. Okinawa's status as a longevity hotspot is now threatened as the population following traditional dietary patterns literally dies out [59].

This natural experiment provides compelling evidence that Okinawan longevity wasn't genetic. It was dietary. Change the diet, and the health advantages disappear within a single generation.

Common Patterns Across Blue Zones

Despite geographic and cultural differences, Blue Zone diets share consistent patterns that align with the principles outlined in this book.

Plant-Predominant, Not Plant-Exclusive

Blue Zone diets derive approximately 90-95% of calories from plants: vegetables, fruits, legumes, whole grains, and nuts. Animal products are consumed, but as condiments or small portions rather than centerpieces. This represents a dramatic inversion of the modern Western plate, where meat dominates and vegetables serve as garnish.

Beans as Dietary Cornerstone

Every Blue Zone population consumes beans or legumes as dietary staples. Black beans in Costa Rica, lentils in the Mediterranean, soybeans in Okinawa. These provide protein, fiber, and complex carbohydrates in forms that promote stable blood sugar and healthy gut bacteria.

Whole Grains, Not Refined

When grains are consumed in Blue Zones, they're whole or minimally processed. Traditional sourdough breads, whole oats, brown rice. The refining processes that strip fiber and nutrients from modern grain products are absent from these traditional patterns.

Abundant Vegetables

Blue Zone populations consume five to ten servings of vegetables daily, far exceeding recommendations and dramatically exceeding actual consumption in Western populations. These vegetables are typically local, seasonal, and prepared simply.

Nuts Daily

Most Blue Zone populations consume approximately one to two ounces of nuts daily, typically tree nuts like almonds, walnuts, or cashews. This consistent pattern across geographically diverse populations suggests nuts provide significant health benefits [147].

Meat as Condiment

When meat is consumed in Blue Zones, it's typically in small quantities, often as flavoring rather than the main dish. And it's always from traditionally raised animals eating their natural diets, not industrial CAFO products.

Walter's Return to Roots

Walter, 65, was a retired engineer who had spent his career solving complex problems. When his health began declining in his late fifties, he approached it the same way he approached engineering challenges: with systematic analysis and data.

'I gathered every piece of research I could find on longevity,' he explained. 'I expected to find some complex intervention, some sophisticated supplement protocol, some cutting-edge treatment. Instead, I found Blue Zones. People live longer and healthier than anyone else by eating the simplest possible diet.'

Walter's transition was not about deprivation. It was about simplification. He eliminated processed foods, reduced his meat consumption, dramatically increased his vegetable intake, and started eating beans almost daily. He returned to the dietary patterns his Italian grandmother had followed before her family adopted American eating habits.

'My grandmother lived to 97 and was sharp until the end,' Walter noted. 'My father, who ate American food his whole life, died of heart disease at 68. The data was right in my own family. I just needed to pay attention to it.'

At 65, Walter's inflammatory markers improved dramatically. His need for blood pressure medication had disappeared. His energy levels rivaled those of much younger men. 'I'm not following a diet,' he said. 'I'm just eating what humans ate before we started engineering our food supply [238].'

Applying Blue Zone Principles

You do not need to move to Sardinia or Okinawa to benefit from Blue Zone principles. The dietary patterns that produce exceptional longevity can be adopted anywhere [59].

The R.E.S.T.O.R.E. MILA protocol aligns with Blue Zone dietary principles: elimination of inflammatory processed foods, emphasis on whole foods, adequate protein from quality sources, abundant vegetables, and healthy fats. The difference is that Blue Zone populations never needed a protocol because they never adopted the industrial foods that require elimination.

For modern eaters seeking to optimize health and longevity, Blue Zone research provides both validation and inspiration. The path to health isn't through novel interventions or complex supplements. It is through returning to the dietary patterns that supported human health for millennia [299].

Blue Zone populations demonstrate that the right dietary patterns produce remarkable health outcomes, but they also reveal something equally important: their relationship with food is fundamentally different from modern eating culture. Food is fuel, social connection, and cultural tradition, not entertainment, emotional regulation, or identity.

The next chapter explores the psychology of eating: how to shift from viewing food as entertainment to understanding food as fuel, how taste preferences transform with dietary change, and how to avoid the trap of orthorexia where healthy eating itself becomes unhealthy obsession. Understanding the psychological dimension completes the framework for sustainable dietary transformation.

Key Takeaways

Blue Zone populations, the longest-lived, healthiest people on Earth, naturally follow dietary patterns that exclude most or all of the Toxic Nine, not through conscious health decisions but through traditional eating habits unchanged for generations.

These populations demonstrate that exceptional longevity and health span are achievable through simple, whole-food diets without supplements, sophisticated interventions, or nutrition science.

The Okinawan experience proves these health advantages aren't genetic: when traditional diets are abandoned for Western eating patterns, health declines within a single generation.

Consistent patterns across geographically diverse Blue Zones include plant-predominant eating, beans as dietary staples, daily nut consumption, meat as condiment rather than centerpiece, and complete absence of processed foods.

The R.E.S.T.O.R.E. MILA protocol represents a return to these ancestral patterns, validated by both traditional wisdom and modern research as the foundation for optimal health and longevity.

CHAPTER 12

The Psychology of Eating

Catherine had been a social worker for two decades, helping others navigate emotional challenges while ignoring her own relationship with food. At 44, she finally acknowledged what she had long denied: food had become her primary emotional regulation tool. Stressed? Eat. Sad? Eat. Celebrating? Eat. Bored? Eat. Her weight had climbed steadily, but more troubling was the anxiety she felt when food was not available or when circumstances forced her to deviate from eating patterns that had become ritualized comfort.

'I know what I should eat,' she admitted during our first conversation. 'I've read every nutrition book. I understand the science. But knowing and doing are two different things. The moment I'm stressed or upset, all that knowledge disappears, and I find myself eating things I know are destroying my health. Then I feel guilty, which makes me more stressed, which makes me eat more. It's a cycle I can't seem to break.'

Catherine's struggle represents perhaps the most challenging aspect of dietary transformation: the psychological dimension. Understanding what to eat is relatively simple. Actually, eating that way consistently, in a culture that has transformed food into entertainment, comfort, and identity, requires addressing the emotional and cognitive patterns that drive eating behavior.

Food as Entertainment: The Modern Distortion

For most of human history, food served a straightforward purpose: providing the nutrients and energy necessary for survival. Meals were often simple, repetitive, and eaten primarily for sustenance. The idea that eating should be constantly exciting, varied, and pleasurable would have seemed absurd to our ancestors who were simply grateful to have enough.

Modern food culture has transformed this relationship entirely. Food is now entertainment. We 'treat ourselves' with meals. We plan social events around food. We watch cooking shows, read food magazines, and follow food accounts on social media. The food industry spends billions annually on engineering products designed not for nutrition but for maximum pleasure and repeat consumption [51].

This transformation creates expectations that whole, unprocessed food cannot meet. When eating has become entertainment, foods that are simply nutritious seem boring. The person accustomed to hyper-palatable processed foods experiences real, whole food as bland and unsatisfying.

The Taste Transformation

One of the most remarkable phenomena patients experience when following this protocol is the transformation of taste perception. After approximately 30 days of avoiding sugar and processed foods, taste buds literally change. Foods that once seemed bland have become richly flavored. Natural sweetness in vegetables and fruits becomes pronounced.

This transformation reflects basic biology. Taste buds regenerate every 10 to 14 days. New taste buds that develop in the absence of constant sugar bombardment are more sensitive to sweetness and better able to detect subtle flavors in whole foods.

Patients who persist through the initial weeks often describe a genuine shift in food preferences. 'I used to crave donuts,' one patient told me. 'Now the thought of eating one makes me feel slightly ill. I genuinely prefer an apple. I never thought that would happen.' This isn't willpower. It is physiological change.

Paula's Paradigm Shift

Paula, 51, worked as an executive assistant and had spent her adult life cycling through diets. She would start with enthusiasm, experience temporary success, then regain the lost weight plus additional pounds when willpower inevitably failed.

'Every diet felt like punishment,' she explained. 'I was constantly thinking about what I couldn't have, counting down until I could eat normally again. No wonder I always failed. Who can sustain punishment indefinitely?'

The shift for Paula came when she stopped viewing this as a diet and started viewing it as simply how she ate now. Not a temporary intervention but a permanent change in her relationship with food.

'When I stopped thinking about when I could go back to my old eating,' she said, 'everything changed. There was no going back. This was just how I ate now. Somehow that made it easier, not harder.'

Food as Fuel: The Paradigm Shift

The most successful patients make a fundamental cognitive shift: from viewing food as entertainment to understanding food as fuel. This is not about eliminating pleasure from eating. It is about changing the primary framework through which food is understood.

When food is entertainment, meals need to be exciting. Repetition feels boring. And the constant quest for novel taste experiences leads inevitably toward processed foods engineered for maximum stimulation.

When food is fuel, different criteria apply. The question becomes not 'what do I feel like eating?' but 'what does my body need?' Repetition is fine because fuel doesn't need to be exciting. Simple meals become acceptable because their purpose is nourishment.

Many patients find this shift profoundly liberating. 'I used to spend so much mental energy thinking about food,' one patient observed. 'Now I eat basically the same things most days, and I never think about food between meals. That mental freedom is worth more than any flavor experience.'

Emotional Eating: Understanding the Pattern

For many people, food serves functions far beyond nutrition. It soothes emotional distress. It provides comfort during challenging times. It fills emotional voids that have nothing to do with physical hunger.

Understanding the difference between physical and emotional hunger is crucial. Physical hunger develops gradually, can wait, is satisfied by eating, doesn't trigger guilt, and is located in the stomach. Emotional hunger appears suddenly, feels urgent, persists after eating, often triggers guilt, and is located in the mind [215].

Addressing emotional eating requires developing alternative coping strategies for the emotional needs food has been serving. Identify triggers. Develop alternatives. Create space between trigger and response. Seek support when needed.

Raymond's Recognition

Raymond, 48, worked in IT management, a stressful role that he had navigated for years using food as his primary stress relief.

Late nights at the office meant fast food. Difficult projects meant comfort food.

'I never thought of myself as an emotional eater,' he admitted. 'But when I actually tracked my eating, I realized I was never eating because I was hungry. I was eating because I was stressed, or frustrated, or exhausted.'

Raymond's breakthrough came when he started addressing the underlying issues rather than feeding them. He implemented boundaries around work hours. He began walking during stressful moments rather than reaching for snacks.

'The eating was a symptom, not the problem,' he reflected. 'Once I started actually dealing with the stress instead of eating it, the compulsive eating just stopped.'

The Orthorexia Warning

While most patients struggle with eating too much of the wrong foods, a smaller group develops the opposite problem: an obsessive preoccupation with 'pure' or 'healthy' eating that itself becomes pathological. This condition, called orthorexia nervosa, represents healthy eating taken to an unhealthy extreme [256].

Signs of orthorexia include spending excessive time planning 'pure' foods, experiencing significant anxiety when unable to eat 'correctly,' progressively eliminating food groups beyond what evidence supports, and self-worth becoming tied to dietary compliance [256].

The protocol described in this book is designed to improve health, not to become an identity or source of anxiety. Food should serve life, not dominate it. If following dietary guidelines creates more stress than it resolves, the approach itself has become a problem.

Practical Strategies for Psychological Success

Focus on addition before subtraction. Rather than emphasizing what you're removing, focus on what you're adding: more vegetables, better proteins, healthier fats. Abundance feels better than restriction.

Prepare for the transition period. The first two to four weeks often include cravings, mood fluctuations, and moments of doubt. Understanding this as temporary prevents interpreting these experiences as signs of failure.

Build identity around the change. Rather than 'trying a diet,' become 'someone who eats real food.' Identity-based change is more durable than willpower-based change.

Forgive imperfection. Occasional deviations do not erase progress. Treating them as catastrophes often triggers more significant relapses than the deviation itself.

Catherine's Transformation

Remember Catherine, the social worker whose emotional eating had trapped her in cycles of stress and shame? Her transformation required addressing the psychological dimension as seriously as the nutritional one.

She began therapy focused on stress management and emotional regulation. She developed a toolkit of non-food responses to emotional triggers. She gave herself permission to feel difficult emotions without immediately trying to eat them away.

'The biggest change wasn't in what I ate,' Catherine reflected six months later. 'It was in how I related to food. Food became just food again, not my therapist, not my entertainment, not my reward system. Just fuel for my body. That shift changed everything.'

The psychological dimension of eating connects directly to the practical challenges patients face when implementing this protocol. Questions arise, obstacles appear, and unexpected situations require navigation.

The next chapter addresses the most common questions and troubleshooting challenges: what to do when progress stalls, how to handle family members who eat differently, strategies for limited budgets and time, and guidance for knowing when the protocol can be relaxed and when strictness remains essential.

Key Takeaways

Modern food culture has transformed eating from simple fueling into entertainment, comfort, and identity, creating expectations that whole foods cannot meet and driving consumption of hyper-palatable processed products.

The taste transformation that occurs after approximately 30 days of healthy eating changes both physiological taste bud sensitivity and neurological reward pathways, making healthier foods genuinely more enjoyable.

Emotional eating, driven by stress, loneliness, boredom, or anxiety rather than physical hunger, requires developing alternative coping strategies rather than relying on willpower alone.

The shift from 'food as entertainment' to 'food as fuel' liberates mental energy, reduces food preoccupation, and makes sustainable eating patterns possible.

Orthorexia, the obsessive pursuit of dietary purity, represents healthy eating taken to unhealthy extremes.

Success requires addressing the psychological dimension as seriously as the nutritional one.

CHAPTER 13

Common Questions and Troubleshooting

Eleanor arrived at our follow-up appointment with a notebook full of questions. At 56, this school administrator had been following the protocol for three months with significant improvements in her energy, joint pain, and digestive issues. But as the initial enthusiasm settled into the routine of daily life, practical questions had accumulated.

'I understand the principles,' she said, flipping through her notes. 'But I keep encountering situations where I'm not sure what to do. When can I be flexible? When do I need to be strict? What do I do when my progress stalls? How do I handle my husband who thinks this is all nonsense?'

Eleanor's questions reflected the reality that dietary change doesn't happen in a vacuum. Real life presents complications, obstacles, and situations that simple rules don't address. This chapter provides practical answers to the questions patients most commonly ask.

When Can I Stop Being So Strict?

This question arises frequently, usually around the three-to-six-month mark. Patients who have experienced significant improvement wonder whether they can relax their adherence to the protocol.

The answer depends on several factors. First, what are you actually asking? If you're asking whether you can occasionally deviate without catastrophic consequences, the answer is yes, within the six-times-per-year guideline discussed in Chapter 8. If you're asking whether you can return to regularly eating inflammatory foods, the answer is no.

The Toxic Nine aren't problematic because you're currently unwell. They're problematic because they damage human physiology. A person who has healed doesn't suddenly become immune to the effects of sugar, seed oils, or processed foods. Continued avoidance isn't temporary treatment; it's the way humans should eat for optimal health.

That said, some flexibility becomes possible as health stabilizes. The occasional exposure that might have triggered significant symptoms early in healing may be better tolerated once the gut has healed and inflammatory markers have normalized. The key is recognizing that flexibility means occasional deviation, not return to previous patterns.

Harold's Question About Strictness

Harold, 61, was a consultant who had followed the protocol strictly for eight months. His results had been dramatic: 45 pounds lost, blood pressure normalized, chronic fatigue resolved. He wondered whether he could now be less vigilant.

'I've proven I can do this,' he said. 'Do I really need to be this careful forever?'

We discussed the difference between healing strictness and maintenance flexibility. During active healing, strict adherence accelerates progress and prevents setbacks. Once health has stabilized, some flexibility is possible without losing ground.

For Harold, this meant he could occasionally enjoy a meal at a restaurant without interrogating the server about every ingredient. He could attend social events without bringing his own food. He could use his strategic cheats without anxiety. What it didn't mean was adding seed oils back to his kitchen, resuming regular bread consumption, or returning to processed foods as dietary staples.

'Think of it like brushing your teeth,' I suggested. 'You don't stop because your teeth are healthy. You maintain the practice that created health. But you also don't panic if you miss one brushing while traveling.'

What If My Progress Stalls?

Weight loss plateaus and symptom improvement stalls are common experiences, usually occurring somewhere between weeks four and twelve of the protocol. Patients who were losing weight steadily suddenly stopped. Symptoms that were improving level off. Frustration sets in.

Several factors commonly contribute to stalls

Hidden sources of inflammatory foods. Careful review often reveals ingredients sneaking into the diet through sauces, seasonings, or foods assumed to be compliant. Reading labels more carefully identifies the culprit.

Portion drift. Over time, portions often increase without conscious awareness. Returning to measured portions, particularly of carbohydrates and proteins, often restarts progress.

Inadequate sleep. Sleep deprivation increases cortisol, promotes insulin resistance, and increases hunger hormones. Prioritizing seven to eight hours often breaks plateaus that dietary changes alone could not address.

Insufficient physical activity. While diet creates the foundation, movement accelerates progress. Adding or increasing exercise often restarts stalled progress.

Stress. Chronic stress elevates cortisol, which promotes fat storage, particularly around the midsection. Addressing stress through management techniques may be necessary for continued progress.

Normal metabolic adaptation. After sustaining weight loss, metabolism adjusts. This is normal physiology, not failure. Patience, continued compliance, and sometimes strategic adjustments to caloric intake are appropriate responses.

Melissa's Troubleshooting

Melissa, 43, was a physician who understood the science but was frustrated by her stalled progress. After initial success, her weight loss had stopped, and her energy improvements had plateaued.

Review of her food diary revealed the problem: while she had eliminated the obvious sources of inflammatory foods, hidden sources had crept in. The 'healthy' salad dressing she had been using contained soybean oil. The rotisserie chicken from the grocery store was cooked in seed oils. The 'natural' seasoning blend contained corn derivatives.

'I'm a doctor,' she said, shaking her head. 'I should have caught this.'

Nobody catches everything initially. The food industry is sophisticated at hiding problematic ingredients under acceptable-sounding names. Melissa's progress resumed once she identified and eliminated these hidden sources.

How Do I Handle Family Resistance?

Many patients face resistance from family members who don't share their dietary goals. Spouses may resent changes to shared meals. Children may refuse 'healthy' food. Extended family may view dietary restrictions as personal rejection.

Several strategies help navigate family challenges

Don't make it about them. Your dietary choices are about your health, not judgment of their choices. Communicate this clearly and repeatedly until it's understood.

Cook meals that work for everyone with easy modifications. Serve grilled chicken, rice, and vegetables as the base. Family members who want bread, cheese, or sauces can add them. You eat the base; they customize.

Focus on what you are eating, not what you're avoiding. Enthusiasm about delicious whole foods is more appealing than lectures about what is wrong with processed foods.

Lead by example. As your health improves visibly, curiosity often develops. Many patients report family members gradually adopting aspects of the protocol after seeing results.

Respect their autonomy. You cannot force dietary change on others, nor should you try. Your responsibility is your own health. Their choices belong to them.

What About Budget Constraints?

'This diet is too expensive' is a common objection that deserves serious engagement. Yes, pasture-raised eggs cost more than conventional eggs. Grass-fed beef costs more than grain-fed. Organic produce costs more than conventional.

But the cost comparison is incomplete without considering what you are no longer buying. Processed foods, snack foods, sugary drinks, restaurant meals, the costs add up. Many patients find their food spending stays constant or even decreases despite higher per-item costs for quality ingredients.

Prioritize strategically. If budget is limited, prioritize upgrades that matter most: eggs, then beef and dairy, then chicken and produce.

Buy in bulk. Warehouse stores offer grass-fed beef at prices competitive with conventional grocery store meat. Buying larger quantities and freezing reduces per-unit costs.

Embrace cheaper protein sources. Beans and legumes are extraordinarily inexpensive and provide excellent nutrition. Eggs remain affordable even in pasture-raised form. These can replace more expensive meats at some meals.

Buy frozen vegetables. Frozen vegetables are nutritionally comparable to fresh at significantly lower cost. They also reduce waste since they don't spoil before use.

Consider the true cost. The few dollars extra spent on quality food is cheap compared to medications, doctor visits, lost productivity, and reduced quality of life from diet-related illness. Food quality is healthcare spending in its most effective form.

I Don't Have Time to Cook

Modern life is genuinely busy. Between work, family, and other obligations, many people feel they simply cannot add food preparation to their responsibilities.

Yet consider you don't have time not to eat well. The hours lost to low energy, the days spent sick, the years taken from your life by chronic disease, these costs dwarf time spent preparing food.

Simple meals do not require extensive preparation. Scrambled eggs with vegetables: 10 minutes. Grilled chicken with steamed broccoli: 25 minutes. Fish with roasted vegetables on a sheet pan: 30 minutes including prep. These are not gourmet projects; they're basic fuel preparation.

Batch cooking transforms the equation. Two to three hours once weekly can prepare food for multiple days. Cook six chicken breasts, not one. Bake multiple sweet potatoes. Prepare a large pot of rice. Portion into containers. Meals become assembly, not cooking.

Slow cookers eliminate active cooking time. Add ingredients before work; dinner is ready when you return. No standing over a stove required.

Prioritize ruthlessly. Most people who 'don't have time' to cook find time for television, social media, or other activities that could be reduced. It is about priority, not possibility.

What About Special Populations?

Children

Children can follow this protocol with appropriate age modifications. Focus on addition rather than restriction, emphasizing abundant vegetables, quality proteins, and fruit. Avoid making food a battleground; repeated exposure to healthy foods eventually produces acceptance. Don't create separate 'kid food' categories; children who eat what adults eat develop broader palates.

Pregnant and Nursing Women

This protocol is appropriate for pregnancy and nursing with emphasis on adequate nutrition rather than restriction. Ensure sufficient calories, protein, iron, and folate. Avoid aggressive elimination that could compromise nutritional intake. Consult with healthcare providers regarding individual needs [300].

Athletes and High-Activity Individuals

Higher activity levels require higher caloric intake, particularly carbohydrates. Increase portions of approved carbohydrate sources (sweet potatoes, rice, oatmeal, beans) to match energy expenditure. Timing carbohydrates around activity can improve performance. The fundamental principles remain sound; only quantities adjust.

Elderly

Older adults may need modifications for digestibility and dental issues. Emphasize easy-to-chew proteins, well-cooked vegetables, and softer carbohydrate sources. Ensure adequate protein intake to maintain muscle mass. Address any swallowing difficulties with appropriate food textures.

How Do I Know If This Is Working?

Beyond the scale, multiple indicators suggest the protocol is producing positive changes:

- Energy levels stabilize and improve, particularly elimination of afternoon crashes. Morning energy comes more easily.

- Sleep quality improves. Falling asleep becomes easier, staying asleep more consistent, waking more refreshed.

- Digestive function normalizes. Bloating decreases, bowel movements become regular, discomfort resolves.
- Inflammation markers decrease. Joint pain diminishes, headaches become less frequent, skin conditions improve.
- Mental clarity increases. Brain fog lifts, concentration improves, memory sharpens.
- Mood stabilizes. Anxiety decreases, depression lifts, emotional regulation improves.

These changes often preceded significant weight loss and may be more important indicators of healing than scale movement.

When Should I Seek Additional Help?

This protocol provides foundational nutrition that benefits virtually everyone. However, some situations require additional support:

If symptoms persist despite faithful adherence for three months, further investigation may be needed. Testing through the Dynamic Intake at restoremila.com can help identify additional factors affecting your health.

If you have existing medical conditions requiring medication, work with your healthcare provider as the protocol may reduce medication needs over time.

If you're experiencing emotional eating patterns you cannot address alone, professional support from a therapist specializing in food relationships may be valuable.

If you suspect food sensitivities beyond the Toxic Nine, formal testing can identify individual triggers.

Eleanor's Progress

Eleanor, who opened this chapter with her notebook full of questions, found answers that transformed her experience of the protocol. Understanding when flexibility was appropriate reduced her anxiety. Identifying hidden seed oils in her cooking broke a weight loss plateau. Strategies for navigating her skeptical husband improved family dynamics.

'I was trying to follow perfect rules in an imperfect world,' she reflected. 'Once I understood the principles deeply enough to make judgment calls, everything became easier. It stopped feeling like a diet I was following and started feeling like just how I eat now.'

The questions addressed in this chapter arise naturally during the journey from understanding to implementation. But the most profound transformation lies not in answering specific questions but in experiencing the cumulative effect of consistent whole-food eating.

In conclusion, we return to Maria, whose story opened this book, to witness what eighteen months of commitment to these principles has produced, not just in symptom resolution but in her entire relationship with food, health, and possibility.

Key Takeaways

Strict adherence during active healing transitions to maintained flexibility once health stabilizes.

Return to previous eating patterns remains incompatible with sustained wellness.

Progress stalls commonly result from hidden inflammatory foods, portion drift, inadequate sleep, insufficient activity, or chronic stress, all of which are addressable within the protocol.

Family resistance requires patient leadership by example rather than evangelism, with focus on your own health journey rather than converting others.

Budget constraints can be managed through strategic prioritization, bulk purchasing, cheaper protein sources like eggs and legumes, and recognition that food quality spending replaces medical spending.

Time constraints respond to simple meals, batch cooking, and prioritization of health over optional activities. Signs of success include stable energy, improved sleep, better digestion, reduced inflammation, mental clarity, and mood stability.

The Dynamic Intake at restoremila.com provides personalized guidance when additional support is needed.

CONCLUSION

Your Path Forward

Eighteen months had passed since Maria first walked into my office carrying the weight of fifteen years of suffering. The elementary school teacher who had arrived exhausted, inflamed, and despairing had become someone else entirely, not a different person, but the person she was always meant to be before modern food began dismantling her health.

'I almost canceled that first appointment,' she admitted as we reviewed her progress. 'I have seen so many doctors, tried so many diets, failed so many times. Part of me had given up believing anything could actually help.'

The woman sitting across from me now bore little resemblance to that desperate patient. At 53, Maria had more energy than she remembered having in decades. The brain fog that had made her question her competence as a teacher had completely lifted. The joint pain that had made mornings miserable had resolved. The digestive issues that had ruled her life had normalized. Her chronic fatigue, fibromyalgia, and IBS diagnoses had essentially become historical footnotes.

But the transformation extended beyond symptom resolution. Maria had fundamentally changed her relationship with food, health, and her own body.

Beyond Symptom Resolution

'The symptoms going away were wonderful,' Maria said. 'But that's not actually the biggest change. The biggest change is that I understand my body now. I know why I was sick. I know why I got better. And I know how to stay well.'

This understanding represented something more valuable than any treatment that could provide empowerment. Maria was no longer a passive recipient of diagnoses and prescriptions. She understood the MILA system, the Mitochondrial-Immune-Lymphatic Axis that governs so much of human health. She understood why the Toxic Nine had been destroying that system. And she understood how whole foods, carefully chosen and prepared, supported her body's innate capacity to heal [301].

'When I eat something that doesn't serve me now,' she continued, 'I feel it. Not just vaguely unwell, but specifically. I can identify which system is being stressed. That feedback loop makes the right choices obvious. I don't need willpower because my body tells me clearly what it needs.'

The Ripple Effects

Maria's transformation had not occurred in isolation. Her husband, initially skeptical, had watched her improvement with growing curiosity. After six months of observing her energy surge while his own continued declining, he asked to try the protocol. His blood pressure, previously requiring medication, had normalized within three months of adopting the same principles.

Her two adult children, raised on the same processed foods that had damaged her health, had begun questioning their own dietary patterns. Her daughter, experiencing early signs of the same issues that had plagued Maria, started implementing changes and reported significant improvement. Her son, a former skeptic, had begun reading about nutrition after witnessing his mother's transformation.

'I used to think I was just unlucky,' Maria reflected. 'Bad genes, predisposed to illness, nothing to be done. Now I understand that most of what I suffered was created by what I was eating. That's actually good news because food is something I can control. My health isn't determined by fate. It's determined by choices [238].'

The R.E.S.T.O.R.E. MILA Framework Revisited

Maria's journey had followed the R.E.S.T.O.R.E. MILA framework that provides structure for healing:

Reveal: Through the Dynamic Intake assessment and subsequent testing, we identified the patterns of dysfunction driving her symptoms. Her gut was severely compromised, her inflammatory markers were elevated, and her nutritional status showed significant deficiencies despite what she had believed was healthy eating.

Eliminate: The Toxic Nine, sugar, wheat, corn, soy, dairy, peanuts, seed oils, alcohol, and chemical additives, were systematically removed from her diet. This created the foundation for healing by stopping the ongoing damage.

Strengthen: With the inflammatory burden reduced, her immune system began rebalancing. The chronic activation that had kept her in a state of perpetual inflammation started resolving.

Turbocharge: As her terrain improved, targeted support for mitochondrial function accelerated her recovery. Energy that had been suppressed for years began returning.

Optimize: Fine-tuning her approach based on her individual responses and test results personalized the protocol for her specific needs.

Repair: The damaged systems, gut lining, cellular membranes, detoxification pathways, underwent restoration as the conditions for healing were maintained.

Everlasting Health: The final phase transitions patients from active treatment to maintenance. Ongoing lifestyle practices, seasonal drainage resets, and continued MILA awareness sustain long-term resilience and prevent relapses.

What This Means for You

Maria's story is not unique. Thousands of patients following these principles have experienced similar transformations. The human body has remarkable capacity for healing when given the proper conditions. The problem is that modern food environments create exactly the opposite conditions.

You now possess the knowledge that Maria lacked when her health first began declining. You understand why modern food causes modern disease. You understand the Toxic Nine and why they must be avoided. You understand what whole foods to eat and how to structure your eating. You understand how to navigate real-world challenges. You understand the psychology of sustainable change.

The question is no longer what to do. The question is whether you will do it.

The Choice Before You

Every meal presents a choice. You can choose foods that heal or foods that harm. You can choose to invest a few extra dollars and minutes in quality or accept the consequences of convenience. You can choose to prioritize your long-term health or succumb to short-term pleasure.

These choices compound. A single meal matters little. But thousands of meals, accumulated over years and decades, determine whether you arrive at your later years vibrant and capable or diminished and dependent.

The patients who transform their health share one characteristic: they make a decision and then defend it against the inevitable challenges. They don't engage in endless internal debate about whether to follow the protocol. They simply follow it, treating it as the non-negotiable foundation of their lives.

This isn't about perfection. It's about direction. The occasional deviation doesn't derail a fundamentally sound approach. But chronic ambivalence, perpetually questioning whether to eat well or not, exhausts willpower and produces inferior results.

Your Next Steps

If you're ready to begin your own transformation, the path forward is clear:

First, take the Dynamic Intake assessment at restoremila.com. This comprehensive evaluation will identify your specific patterns of dysfunction and provide personalized recommendations for your unique situation. The assessment adapts to your responses, creating a customized roadmap for your healing journey.

Second, commit to eliminating the Toxic Nine for a minimum of 90 days. This isn't arbitrary; it's the time required for significant healing to occur and for your body to demonstrate what's possible when the inflammatory burden is removed.

Third, follow the eating structure outlined in this book: whole proteins, complex carbohydrates, abundant vegetables, healthy fats, properly timed within your eating window. Use the portion guidelines as starting points and adjust based on your energy and results.

Fourth, prepare for the challenges. Meal prep, restaurant strategies, social navigation, and all the practical skills discussed in this book will be needed. Don't wait for problems to arise; anticipate them with solutions already in place.

Fifth, track your progress beyond the scale. Energy levels, sleep quality, digestive function, mental clarity, joint comfort, all of these provide feedback about how your body is responding. Celebrate improvements in these areas; they often precede weight changes.

Support is Available

You don't have to navigate this journey alone. At restoremila.com, you'll find resources designed to support your transformation:

- The Dynamic Intake assessment provides personalized analysis of your health patterns and specific recommendations for your situation.

- Supplement recommendations, carefully vetted for quality and efficacy, address the specific needs identified through your assessment.
- Ongoing education keeps you informed about the latest understanding of nutrition and health.
- Community connection provides support from others on similar journeys.

The investment in the Dynamic Intake is reimbursed with your first purchase, reflecting our confidence that once you understand your unique patterns, you'll want the targeted support that accelerates healing.

Maria's Final Words

As our appointment concluded, Maria offered advice for anyone beginning this journey:

'Don't wait until you're as sick as I was. I wish I had understood this twenty years ago. But also, don't despair if you're already suffering. I was told my conditions were chronic and incurable. They weren't. They were my body's response to what I was eating, and when I changed what I ate, my body healed.'

She paused, choosing her next words carefully.

'The hardest part was the first three weeks. My body was addicted to the foods that were destroying it, and withdrawal was uncomfortable. But once I pushed through that period, everything changed. The foods I once couldn't live without lost their appeal. The foods I thought were boring became delicious. My taste buds literally transformed.'

'Now I can't imagine going back. Not because I'm depriving myself, but because I genuinely prefer how I eat now. I prefer how I feel. I prefer being the person who can walk up stairs without getting winded, who doesn't need to nap every afternoon, who can think clearly and remember names and participate fully in life.'

Maria stood to leave, the same teacher who had walked in eighteen months earlier yet utterly transformed.

'This isn't a diet,' she said at the door. 'It's just how humans are supposed to eat. Once you understand that, everything else falls into place.'

Your Story Begins Now

Maria's story has reached its current chapter, but yours is just beginning. The principles in this book have transformed lives. They have resolved conditions that conventional medicine declared incurable. They have restored energy, clarity, and joy that people thought were lost forever.

These principles work not because they are novel or extreme, but because they align with human biology. Your body wants to heal. It's designed to heal. The problem isn't that healing is impossible. The problem is that modern food creates conditions where healing cannot occur.

Remove the obstacles. Provide the raw materials. Follow the sequence. And your body will do what bodies have done for hundreds of thousands of years: restore itself to the state of health it was designed to maintain.

The food revolution your body has been waiting for starts with your next meal.

Start now.

Visit restoremila.com to take your Dynamic Intake and begin your personalized journey to restored health.

Key Takeaways

Maria's eighteen-month transformation from chronic illness to vibrant health demonstrates that conditions conventionally labeled as permanent can resolve when their root cause, inflammatory modern food, is addressed.

Understanding the MILA system and the Toxic Nine empowers patients to become active participants in their health rather than passive recipients of diagnoses and medications.

The R.E.S.T.O.R.E. framework provides structured progression from revealing dysfunction through restoring optimal function.

Transformation requires decision followed by consistent action rather than perpetual deliberation about whether to follow the protocol.

The Dynamic Intake at restoremila.com provides personalized assessment and recommendations that accelerate and optimize the healing journey.

This approach isn't a temporary diet but a return to the eating patterns that human biology requires, and once understood and experienced, most patients cannot imagine returning to the foods that caused their suffering.

Ready to begin? Scan the code below to complete Dr. Thoma's Dynamic Intake and receive a personalized roadmap for your R.E.S.T.O.R.E. *MILA journey.*

Glossary

A

Acidosis

A condition where the stomach or body fluids become too acidic, causing pain and damage to tissues. In cattle, this occurs when they eat too much grain instead of grass.

Anaphylaxis

A severe, life-threatening allergic reaction that can occur within minutes of exposure to an allergen. Symptoms may include difficulty breathing, swelling, and rapid drop in blood pressure.

Antibodies

Proteins made by the immune system to identify and fight off harmful substances like bacteria, viruses, or foods the body perceives as threats.

Antibiotic Resistance

When bacteria adapt and become immune to antibiotics, it makes infections harder to treat. This happens when antibiotics are overused, especially in animal agriculture.

ATP (Adenosine Triphosphate)

The energy currency of cells. Mitochondria produce ATP, which powers all biological processes in the body. Low ATP production leads to fatigue and cellular dysfunction.

Autoimmune/Autoimmunity

When the immune system mistakenly attacks the body's own healthy tissues. Examples include rheumatoid arthritis, Hashimoto's thyroiditis, and lupus. Often triggered by chronic inflammation from poor diet.

B

Beta-Carotene

An orange pigment found in plants that the body converts into vitamin A. It gives carrots and sweet potatoes their orange color and is important for eye health and immune function.

Bioaccumulation

The process is where toxins, chemicals, and pollutants build up in an animal's fat tissue over time. When we eat that animal, we consume those concentrated toxins.

Blue Zones

Five regions around the world where people regularly live past 100 years old in good health. These areas include Okinawa (Japan), Sardinia (Italy), Nicoya Peninsula (Costa Rica), Ikaria (Greece), and Loma Linda (California).

C

CAFO (Concentrated Animal Feeding Operation)

Large-scale industrial farms where thousands of animals are confined in small spaces, fed unnatural diets, and given antibiotics to prevent disease. Over 95% of U.S. meat comes from CAFOs.

Carotenoids

Natural pigments found in plants that give fruits and vegetables their red, orange, and yellow colors. They act as antioxidants and support immune health.

CDR (Cell Danger Response)

A protective state where mitochondria shift from energy production to defense mode when they detect threats like toxins or infections. Meant to be temporary, but modern inflammatory foods keep cells locked in this danger mode, leading to chronic fatigue and disease.

Centenarians

People who live to be 100 years old or older. Blue Zone regions have unusually high concentrations of healthy centenarians.

Chronic Disease

Long-lasting health conditions that persist for months or years, such as diabetes, heart disease, autoimmune disorders, and obesity. Most chronic diseases are driven by chronic inflammation from poor diet.

Cortisol

A hormone released by the body in response to stress. While helpful in short bursts, chronically elevated cortisol from ongoing stress promotes fat storage, disrupts sleep, and weakens the immune system.

CLA (Conjugated Linoleic Acid)
A beneficial fatty acid found in grass-fed beef and dairy that helps reduce inflammation and improve body composition. Grain-fed animals contain much less CLA.

CRP (C-Reactive Protein)
A protein in the blood that rises when there is inflammation in the body. High CRP levels indicate chronic inflammation and increased disease risk.

D

Dioxins
Toxic chemical pollutants that accumulate in animal fat and can cause cancer and hormone disruption in humans who consume contaminated animal products.

Dynamic Intake
A comprehensive health assessment available at restoremila.com that identifies patterns of dysfunction and provides personal recommendations for healing.

E

Enzyme Deficiency
A condition where the body lacks specific enzymes needed to properly digest certain foods. Lactose intolerance is a

common example where the enzyme lactase is missing or insufficient.

Enzyme Inhibitors

Compounds found in some foods (especially soy and raw grains) that block the enzymes needed to digest protein and nutrients, leading to poor absorption and digestive problems.

Estrogen

A primary female sex hormone that regulates reproduction and many other body functions. Hormone-treated meat and dairy can contain excess estrogen that disrupts human hormone balance.

F

Fermentation

A process where beneficial bacteria or yeast breaks down food, making it easier to digest and creating beneficial compounds. Examples include sourdough bread, yogurt, and miso.

Fibromyalgia

A chronic condition causing widespread muscle pain, fatigue, and sleep problems. Often improves dramatically with dietary changes that reduce inflammation.

FODMAPs

Fermentable Oligosaccharides, Disaccharides, Monosaccharides, and Polyols. These are types of carbohydrates that can cause digestive symptoms in sensitive individuals because they ferment in the gut.

G

Goiter

An enlargement of the thyroid gland that causes a visible swelling in the neck. It can be caused by iodine deficiency or by goitrogenic foods that block iodine absorption.

Goitrogenic Compounds

Substances found in soy and some other foods that interfere with the thyroid gland's ability to absorb iodine, potentially leading to hypothyroidism and goiter.

Grass-Fed

Refers to animals (usually cattle) raised eating only grass and forage, their natural diet. Grass-fed meat has better fatty acid ratios and higher nutrient content than grain-fed meat.

Gut Barrier

The protective lining of the intestines that controls what passes from food into the bloodstream. When damaged (leaky gut), it allows toxins and undigested food particles to enter the blood, triggering inflammation.

Gynecomastia

Development of breast tissue in men, often caused by hormone imbalances. It can occur from consuming foods with hormone-disrupting compounds like soy isoflavones.

H

Hashimoto's Thyroiditis

An autoimmune disease where the immune system attacks the thyroid gland, leading to hypothyroidism. Often worsened by goitrogenic foods like soy and by chronic inflammation.

HDL (High-Density Lipoprotein)

Often called 'good cholesterol,' HDL carries cholesterol away from arteries back to the liver. Higher HDL levels are associated with better heart health.

Histamine Intolerance

A condition where the body has difficulty processing histamine, a chemical found naturally in certain foods or produced by gut bacteria. This can cause headaches, digestive issues, and skin problems.

Hormone Disruption

When chemicals or compounds interfere with the body's natural hormone production or function. Soy isoflavones, hormones in meat/dairy, and certain food additives can disrupt human hormones.

Hypothyroidism

A condition where the thyroid gland doesn't produce enough thyroid hormones, leading to fatigue, weight gain, and slowed metabolism. Can be caused or worsened by goitrogenic foods.

I

IBS (Irritable Bowel Syndrome)

A common digestive disorder causing abdominal pain, bloating, and changes in bowel habits. Often dramatically improves with elimination of inflammatory foods.

IgE (Immunoglobulin E)

Antibodies that trigger immediate allergic reactions. IgE allergies produce symptoms within minutes to two hours and can be life-threatening (like peanut allergies).

IgG (Immunoglobulin G)

Antibodies that trigger delayed food sensitivities. IgG reactions can occur hours to days after eating, making them difficult to identify without testing.

Inflammation

The body's response to injury or harmful substances. Acute inflammation helps healing, but chronic inflammation from poor diets contributes to most modern diseases.

Insulin

A hormone produced by the pancreas that helps cells absorb sugar (glucose) from the blood. Repeated sugar and refined carb consumption leads to insulin resistance, where cells stop responding properly to insulin.

Insulin Resistance

A condition where cells become less responsive to insulin, requiring the body to produce more and more insulin to manage blood sugar. Leads to Type 2 diabetes, weight gain, and metabolic dysfunction.

Intestinal Permeability (Leaky Gut)

A condition where the lining of the intestines becomes damaged, allowing food particles and toxins to leak into the bloodstream and trigger immune reactions.

L

LDL (Low-Density Lipoprotein)

Often called 'bad cholesterol,' LDL carries cholesterol to arteries. Elevated levels, especially oxidized LDL, increase heart disease risk.

Legumes

A family of plants that includes beans, lentils, peas, and peanuts. Most legumes (except peanuts) are healthy protein and fiber sources featured prominently in Blue Zone diets.

Lymphatic System

The body's drainage and waste removal system that transports toxins, cellular debris, and excess fluid away from tissues. When clogged by inflammation and poor diet, toxins accumulate, causing swelling and disease.

M

MILA (Mitochondrial-Immune-Lymphatic Axis)

The interconnected system of cellular energy production (mitochondria), immune defense, and toxin drainage (lymphatic system). When this axis functions properly, health is maintained. When disrupted by poor diet, disease develops.

Metabolic Dysfunction

When the body's ability to process food and produce energy becomes impaired. Includes conditions like insulin resistance, obesity, and metabolic syndrome. Usually caused by chronic consumption of inflammatory foods.

Mitochondria

Tiny structures inside cells that produce energy. Often called the 'powerhouse of the cell,' healthy mitochondria are essential for energy, metabolism, and overall health.

N

Nightshades

A family of plants including tomatoes, potatoes, eggplants, and peppers. Some people are sensitive to nightshades, though they are not part of the Toxic Nine.

Nixtamalization

A traditional process of treating corn with alkali (like lime water) that improves its nutritional value and makes it easier to digest. Traditional tortillas use this process.

O

Omega-3 Fatty Acids

Essential fats that reduce inflammation, support brain health, and protect the heart. Found in fish, grass-fed meat, and some plants. Modern diets are typically deficient in omega-3s.

Omega-6 Fatty Acids

Essential fats that can promote inflammation when consumed in excess. Modern diets contain too much omega-6 (from seed oils and grain-fed meat), creating unhealthy ratios with omega-3.

Orthorexia

An unhealthy obsession with eating 'pure' or 'healthy' foods that becomes psychologically damaging. Food should serve life, not dominate it.

P

Pasture-Raised

Refers to animals raised outdoors with access to pasture, sunshine, and space to move naturally. Pasture-raised products are nutritionally superior to CAFO products.

PCBs (Polychlorinated Biphenyls)

Toxic industrial chemicals that persist in the environment and accumulate in animal fat. They can cause cancer and disrupt hormones in people who consume contaminated products.

Perimenopause

The transition period before menopause when hormone levels fluctuate, typically occurring in a woman's 40s. Symptoms include hot flashes, mood changes, and irregular periods.

Phytates

Natural compounds in grains and seeds that can bind to minerals and reduce their absorption. Traditional preparation methods like soaking and fermentation reduce phytate content.

Polycystic Ovary Syndrome (PCOS)

A hormonal disorder in women causing irregular periods, excess male hormones, and difficulty conceiving. Often improves significantly with dietary changes.

Progesterone

A female sex hormone important for menstrual cycles and pregnancy. Synthetic versions are sometimes given to cattle to promote growth, and these hormones can remain in meat and affect human health.

R

R.E.S.T.O.R.E. MILA Framework

A structured approach to healing that includes Reveal (identify dysfunction), Eliminate (remove toxins), Strengthen (support immune system), Turbocharge (boost mitochondria), Optimize (personalize approach), Repair (restore damaged systems), and Everlasting Health (maintain long-term wellness).

rBGH (Recombinant Bovine Growth Hormone)

A synthetic hormone given to dairy cows to increase milk production. Hormones remain in the milk and can affect human health, including early puberty and cancer risk.

Rheumatoid Arthritis

An autoimmune disease causing painful inflammation of the joints. Many cases improve significantly when inflammatory foods are eliminated from the diet.

Rumen

The first and largest stomach chamber in cows and other ruminants, designed to ferment and digest grass. Feeding grain instead of grass damages the rumen and causes acidosis.

Ruminants

Animals like cattle, sheep, and goats with specialized multi-chamber stomachs designed to digest grass and other fibrous plants through fermentation.

S

Seed Oils

Highly processed oils extracted from seeds using industrial methods, including soybean, corn, canola, safflower, sunflower, and cottonseed oils. These oils are high in inflammatory omega-6 fatty acids and are part of the Toxic Nine.

T

Terrain-Based Medicine

An approach to health that focuses on creating an internal environment (terrain) where disease cannot thrive, rather than just fighting disease symptoms. Emphasizes nutrition, detoxification, and supporting the body's natural healing capacity.

Testosterone

The primary male sex hormone that regulates muscle mass, bone density, and reproductive function. It can be disrupted by soy isoflavones and hormones in conventional meat and dairy. Also given to cattle to promote growth.

Thyroid Hormones

Hormones produced by the thyroid gland that regulate metabolism, energy production, and body temperature. Production can be disrupted by goitrogenic foods like soy and by chronic inflammation.

Toxic Nine

The nine categories of foods that drive modern chronic disease: sugar, wheat, corn, soy, dairy, peanuts, seed oils, alcohol, and chemical additives. Eliminating these foods creates the foundation for healing.

Trypsin Inhibitors

Compounds found in soy and raw grains that block trypsin, an enzyme needed to digest protein. This leads to poor protein absorption and can trigger immune reactions to undigested protein fragments.

W

Wild-Caught

Fish caught in their natural environment, as opposed to farm raised. Wild-caught fish have better fatty acid profiles and lower levels of pollutants than farmed fish.

Z

Zonulin

A protein that regulates the permeability of the intestinal lining. Elevated zonulin levels indicate increased intestinal permeability (leaky gut). Levels typically normalize when inflammatory foods are eliminated.

Reference

[1] Carney TJ. Advancing chronic disease practice through the integration of data and partnerships. Prev Chronic Dis. 2023;20:230120.

[2] Dinse GE, Parks CG, Weinberg CR, et al. Increasing prevalence of antinuclear antibodies in the United States. Arthritis Rheumatol. 2020;72(6):1026-1035.

[3] Centers for Disease Control and Prevention. Diabetes in young people is on the rise. Updated May 15, 2024.

[4] Nunnari J, Suomalainen A. Mitochondria: In sickness and in health. Cell. 2012;148(6):1145-1159.

[5] Naviaux RK. Cell danger response biology: the new science that connects environmental health with mitochondria and the microbiome. Mitochondrion. 2020;51:40-45.

[6] Miller FW, et al. The increasing prevalence of autoimmunity and autoimmune diseases: an urgent call to action. Curr Opin Immunol. 2022;80:102266.

[7] Kataru RP, et al. Regulation of immune function by the lymphatic system in lymphedema. Front Immunol. 2019;10:470.

[8] USDA Economic Research Service. Sugar and sweeteners yearbook tables. 2022.

[9] Drago S, El Asmar R, Di Pierro M, et al. Gliadin, zonulin and gut permeability: effects on celiac and non-celiac intestinal mucosa. Scand J Gastroenterol. 2006;41(4):408-419.

[10] Igbinedion SO, et al. Non-celiac gluten sensitivity: all wheat attack is not celiac. World J Gastroenterol. 2017;23(40):7201-7210.

[11] USDA ERS. Adoption of genetically engineered crops in the United States: recent trends in GE adoption. Updated Dec 12, 2025.

[12] Brooke-Taylor S, Dwyer K, Woodford K, Kost N. Systematic review of the gastrointestinal effects of A1 compared with A2 beta-casein. Nutrients. 2017;9(2):739.

[13] National Cancer Institute. Aflatoxins. Updated Jul 3, 2024.

[14] Raatz SK, et al. Trends in linoleic acid intake in United States adult men and women. Prostaglandins Leukot Essent Fatty Acids. 2018;132:9-13.

[15] World Health Organization (WHO) Europe. No level of alcohol consumption is safe for our health. Jan 4, 2023.

[16] Marketdata Enterprises. U.S. weight loss market reached $89.9B in 2023; forecast $93.8B in 2024. Mar 6, 2024.

[17] Takashima S, et al. Under stressed conditions, proton pump inhibitors enhance intestinal permeability via dysbiosis. Aliment Pharmacol Ther. 2020;52(3):483-493.

[18] Banach M, Serban C, Sahebkar A, et al. Statin therapy and plasma coenzyme Q10 concentrations: a systematic review and meta-analysis. Mayo Clin Proc. 2015;90(1):24-34.

[19] Fujimori S. What are the effects of non-steroidal anti-inflammatory drugs on the small intestine? World J Gastroenterol. 2009;15(26):3202-3204.

[20] Shewry PR, Hey SJ. The contribution of wheat to human diet and health. Food Energy Secur. 2015;4(3):178-202.

[21] Dubcovsky J, Dvorak J. Genome plasticity a key factor in the success of polyploid wheat under domestication. Science. 2007;316(5833):1862-1866.

[22] Khush GS. Green revolution: preparing for the 21st century. Genome. 1999;42(4):646-655.

[23] Fasano A. Zonulin and its regulation of intestinal barrier function: the biological door to inflammation, autoimmunity, and cancer. Physiol Rev. 2011;91(1):151-175.

[24] Gobbetti M, et al. How the sourdough may affect the functional features of leavened baked goods. Food Microbiol. 2014;37:30-40.

[25] Mintz SW. Sweetness and Power: The Place of Sugar in Modern History. New York: Viking; 1985.

[26] Ng SW, Slining MM, Popkin BM. Use of caloric and noncaloric sweeteners in US consumer packaged foods. J Acad Nutr Diet. 2012;112(11):1828-1834.

[27] Centers for Disease Control and Prevention. National Diabetes Statistics Report, 2024. Atlanta, GA: CDC; 2024.

[28] Younossi ZM, et al. Global epidemiology of nonalcoholic fatty liver disease. Nat Rev Gastroenterol Hepatol. 2018;15(1):11-20.

[29] Brownlee M. Advanced protein glycosylation in diabetes and aging. Annu Rev Med. 1995;46:223-234.

[30] David LA, et al. Diet rapidly and reproducibly alters the human gut microbiome. Nature. 2014;505(7484):559-563.

[31] Sanchez A, et al. Role of sugars in human neutrophilic phagocytosis. Am J Clin Nutr. 1973;26(11):1180-1184.

[32] Avena NM, Rada P, Hoebel BG. Evidence for sugar addiction: behavioral and neurochemical effects of intermittent, excessive sugar intake. Neurosci Biobehav Rev. 2008;32(1):20-39.

[33] Vázquez-Padrón ME, et al. Cry1Ac protoxin from Bacillus thuringiensis binds to surface proteins in the mouse small intestine. Biochem Biophys Res Commun. 2000;271(1):54-58.

[34] Aris A, Leblanc S. Maternal and fetal exposure to pesticides associated to genetically modified foods. Reprod Toxicol. 2011;31(4):528-533.

[35] Benbrook CM. Trends in glyphosate herbicide use in the United States and globally. Environ Sci Eur. 2016;28(1):3.

[36] Benbrook CM. Trends in glyphosate herbicide use in the United States and globally. Environ Sci Eur. 2016;28(1):3.

[37] Myers JP, et al. Concerns over use of glyphosate-based herbicides and risks associated with exposures. Environ Health. 2016;15:19.

[38] Teicholz N. The Big Fat Surprise: Why Butter, Meat and Cheese Belong in a Healthy Diet. New York: Simon & Schuster; 2014.

[39] Keys A. Seven Countries: A Multivariate Analysis of Death and Coronary Heart Disease. Cambridge: Harvard University Press; 1980.

[40] Ramsden CE, et al. Re-evaluation of the traditional diet-heart hypothesis: analysis of recovered data from Minnesota Coronary Experiment. BMJ. 2016;353:i1246.

[41] Blasbalg TL, et al. Changes in consumption of omega-3 and omega-6 fatty acids in the United States during the 20th century. Am J Clin Nutr. 2011;93(5):950-962.

[42] Ramsden CE, et al. Changes in consumption of omega-3 and omega-6 fatty acids in the United States during the 20th century. Am J Clin Nutr. 2011;93(5):950-962.

[43] Burdock GA, Carabin IG. Safety assessment of hexane as a food ingredient. Regul Toxicol Pharmacol. 2007;49(2):78-95.

[44] Simopoulos AP. The importance of the ratio of omega-6/omega-3 essential fatty acids. Biomed Pharmacother. 2002;56(8):365-379.

[45] Niki E. Lipid peroxidation: physiological levels and dual biological effects. Free Radic Biol Med. 2009;47(5):469-484.

[46] Neltner TG, et al. Navigating the U.S. food additive regulatory program. Compr Rev Food Sci Food Saf. 2011;10(6):342-368.

[47] Neltner TG, et al. Conflicts of interest in approvals of additives to food determined to be generally recognized as safe. JAMA Intern Med. 2013;173(22):2032-2036.

[48] Neltner TG, et al. Conflicts of interest in approvals of additives to food determined to be generally recognized as safe. JAMA Intern Med. 2013;173(22):2032-2036.

[49] Chassaing B, et al. Dietary emulsifiers impact the mouse gut microbiota promoting colitis and metabolic syndrome. Nature. 2015;519(7541):92-96.

[50] McCann D, et al. Food additives and hyperactive behaviour in children: a randomised, double-blinded, placebo-controlled trial. Lancet. 2007;370(9598):1560-1567.

[51] Moss M. Salt Sugar Fat: How the Food Giants Hooked Us. New York: Random House; 2013.

[52] Environmental Working Group. Banned in Europe but not the US. EWG Report; 2020.

[53] Chassaing B, et al. Dietary emulsifiers impact the mouse gut microbiota promoting colitis and metabolic syndrome. Nature. 2015;519(7541):92-96.

[54] Pepino MY. Metabolic effects of non-nutritive sweeteners. Physiol Behav. 2015;152:450-455.

[55] Davis DR, et al. Changes in USDA food composition data for 43 garden crops, 1950 to 1999. J Am Coll Nutr. 2004;23(6):669-682.

[56] Kader AA, ed. Postharvest Technology of Horticultural Crops. 3rd ed. University of California ANR Publications; 2002.

[57] Tracy WF. Sweet corn. In: Hallauer AR, ed. Specialty Corns. 2nd ed. Boca Raton: CRC Press; 2001:155-198.

[58] Montgomery DR. Growing a Revolution: Bringing Our Soil Back to Life. New York: W.W. Norton; 2017.

[59] Buettner D, Skemp S. Blue Zones: Lessons from the world's longest lived. Am J Lifestyle Med. 2016;10(5):318-321.

[60] Pes GM, et al. Lifestyle and nutrition related to male longevity in Sardinia: an ecological study. Nutr Metab Cardiovasc Dis. 2013;23(3):212-219.

[61] Willcox DC, et al. The Okinawan diet: health implications of a low-calorie, nutrient-dense, antioxidant-rich dietary pattern. J Am Coll Nutr. 2009;28 Suppl:500S-516S.

[62] Cordain L, et al. Origins and evolution of the Western diet: health implications for the 21st century. Am J Clin Nutr. 2005;81(2):341-354.

[63] Lustig RH. Sugar Has 56 Names: A Shopper's Guide. New York: Penguin Random House; 2013.

[64] Reaven GM. Role of insulin resistance in human disease. Diabetes. 1988;37(12):1595-1607.

[65] Sanchez A, et al. Role of sugars in human neutrophilic phagocytosis. Am J Clin Nutr. 1973;26(11):1180-1184.

[66] De Filippo C, et al. Impact of diet in shaping gut microbiota revealed by a comparative study in children from Europe and rural Africa. Proc Natl Acad Sci USA. 2010;107(33):14691-14696.

[67] Stylianou E, et al. The effect of artificial sweeteners on gut microbiota. Nutrients. 2019;11(10):2285.

[68] Walton RG, et al. Adverse reactions to aspartame. Biol Psychiatry. 1993;34(1):13-17.

[69] Fasano A. Zonulin, regulation of tight junctions, and autoimmune diseases. Ann N Y Acad Sci. 2012;1258(1):25-33.

[70] Feldman M, Richardson CT. Role of thought, sight, smell, and taste of food in the cephalic phase of gastric acid secretion in humans. Gastroenterology. 1986;90(2):428-433.

[71] Fukudome Y, Yoshikawa M. Opioid peptides derived from wheat gluten: their isolation and characterization. FEBS Lett. 1992;296(1):107-111.

[72] Dalla Pellegrina C, et al. Plant lectins as carriers for oral drugs: Is wheat germ agglutinin a suitable candidate? Toxicol Appl Pharmacol. 2005;207(2):170-178.

[73] USDA National Agricultural Statistics Service. Acreage Report. USDA-NASS; June 2023.

[74] Rubio-Infante N, Moreno-Fierros L. An overview of the safety and biological effects of Bacillus thuringiensis Cry toxins in mammals. J Appl Toxicol. 2016;36(5):630-648.

[75] Schlame M, Greenberg ML. Biosynthesis, remodeling and turnover of mitochondrial cardiolipin. Biochim Biophys Acta. 2017;1862(1):3-7.

[76] Tappy L, Le KA. Metabolic effects of fructose and the worldwide increase in obesity. Physiol Rev. 2010;90(1):23-46.

[77] U.S. Department of Agriculture. National Nutrient Database for Standard Reference. USDA Agricultural Research Service; 2023.

[78] Grootveld M, et al. Evidence-based challenges to the continued recommendation and use of peroxidation-susceptible polyunsaturated fatty acid-rich culinary oils. Lipid Technol. 2014;26(7):151-154.

[79] Samsel A, Seneff S. Glyphosate's suppression of cytochrome P450 enzymes and amino acid biosynthesis by the gut microbiome: pathways to modern diseases. Entropy. 2013;15(4):1416-1463.

[80] VandeHaar MJ, St-Pierre N. Major advances in nutrition: relevance to the sustainability of the modern dairy industry. J Dairy Sci. 2006;89(4):1280-1291.

[81] Elliott KB, et al. Beta-casomorphins found in the infant circulation after oral administration of cows milk-derived casein. Peptides. 1984;5(6):1139-1141.

[82] Bell SM, et al. Beta-casomorphins and opioid receptor binding: relationship to physiological effects. Nutr Neurosci. 2006;9(5-6):253-261.

[83] Woodford K. Devil in the Milk: Illness, Health and the Politics of A1 and A2 Milk. White River Junction: Chelsea Green Publishing; 2007.

[84] Hamilton-Reeves JM, et al. Clinical studies show no effects of soy protein or isoflavones on reproductive hormones in men. Fertil Steril. 2010;94(3):997-1007.

[85] Fox PF, McSweeney PLH. Dairy Chemistry and Biochemistry. London: Blackie Academic and Professional; 1998.

[86] Jiang XC, et al. Homogenization of milk alters the physiological properties of fat globule membrane. J Dairy Sci. 2006;89(1):41-50.

[87] Daxenberger A, et al. Possible health impact of animal oestrogens in food. Hum Reprod Update. 2001;7(3):340-355.

[88] Chan JM, et al. Plasma insulin-like growth factor-I and prostate cancer risk: a prospective study. Science. 1998;279(5350):563-566.

[89] Rojas-Rueda PM, et al. Pesticide residues in milk and dairy products. Food Addit Contam Part A. 2015;32(5):657-683.

[90] USDA Economic Research Service. Peanuts: background. 2020.

[91] Bennett JW, Klich M. Mycotoxins. Clin Microbiol Rev. 2003;16(3):497-516.

[92] International Agency for Research on Cancer. IARC Monographs on the Evaluation of Carcinogenic Risks to Humans, vol. 56. Lyon: IARC; 1993.

[93] Turner PC, et al. The role of aflatoxins in the etiology of hepatocellular carcinoma. Annu Rev Pharmacol Toxicol. 2009;49:395-418.

[94] Sharon N, Lis H. Lectins: carbohydrate-specific proteins that mediate cellular recognition. Chem Rev. 1998;98(2):637-674.

[95] USDA National Nutrient Database. Nuts, peanuts, all types, raw. 2019.

[96] Gokmen V, et al. Formation of acrylamide in foods. In: Friedman M, Mottram D, eds. Acrylamide in Food. New York: Springer; 2005:45-68.

[97] Fernandez-Cornejo P, et al. Pesticide use in U.S. agriculture: 21 selected crops, 1960-2008. USDA Economic Research Service; May 2014.

[98] Calder PC. Omega-3 fatty acids and inflammatory processes: from molecules to man. Biochem Soc Trans. 2017;45(5):1105-1115.

[99] Sicherer SH, Sampson HA. Peanut allergy: epidemiology, diagnosis, and management. J Allergy Clin Immunol Pract. 2014;2(6):650-651.

[100] Moss M. The extraordinary science of addictive junk food. New York Times Magazine. Feb 20, 2013.

[101] Simopoulos AP. An increase in the omega-6/omega-3 fatty acid ratio increases the risk for obesity. Nutrients. 2016;8(3):128.

[102] Niki E, et al. Lipid peroxidation: mechanisms, inhibition, and biological effects. Biochem Biophys Res Commun. 2005;338(1):668-676.

[103] Ramsden CE, et al. Dietary linoleic acid and risk of coronary heart disease. Int J Epidemiol. 2014;43(6):1972-1984.

[104] Grootveld M, et al. Health effects of oxidized heated oils. Foodservice Research International. 2001;13(1):41-55.

[105] Grootveld M, et al. In vivo absorption, metabolism, and urinary excretion of alpha,beta-unsaturated aldehydes in experimental animals. Chem Res Toxicol. 1998;11:1176-1183.

[106] Butterfield DA, et al. Roles of amyloid beta-peptide-associated oxidative stress and brain protein modifications in Alzheimer's disease. Free Radic Biol Med. 2002;32(11):1050-1060.

[107] Guillen MD, Goicoechea E. Toxic oxygenated alpha,beta-unsaturated aldehydes and their study in foods. Crit Rev Food Sci Nutr. 2008;48(2):119-136.

[108] Puri P, et al. A lipidomic analysis of nonalcoholic fatty liver disease. Hepatology. 2007;46(4):1081-1090.

[109] Deol P, et al. Soybean oil is more obesogenic and diabetogenic than coconut oil and fructose in mouse. PLoS One. 2015;10(7):e0132672.

[110] Tilg H, Moschen AR. Evolution of inflammation in nonalcoholic fatty liver disease. Gut. 2010;59(12):1536-1544.

[111] Whelan J, Fritsche K. Linoleic acid. Adv Nutr. 2013;4(3):311-312.

[112] GBD 2016 Alcohol Collaborators. Alcohol use and burden for 195 countries and territories, 1990-2016. Lancet. 2018;392:1015-1035.

[113] Stockwell T, et al. Do moderate drinkers have reduced mortality risk? A systematic review and meta-analysis. J Stud Alcohol Drugs. 2016;77(2):185-198.

[114] International Agency for Research on Cancer. Personal habits and indoor combustions. IARC Monographs, vol. 100E. 2012.

[115] Bagnardi V, et al. Alcohol consumption and site-specific cancer risk. Br J Cancer. 2015;112(3):580-593.

[116] Lieber CS. Metabolism of alcohol. Clin Liver Dis. 2005;9(1):1-35.

[117] Seitz HK, Stickel F. Molecular mechanisms of alcohol-mediated carcinogenesis. Nat Rev Cancer. 2007;7(8):599-612.

[118] Das SK, Vasudevan DM. Alcohol-induced oxidative stress. Life Sci. 2007;81(3):177-187.

[119] Manzo-Avalos S, Saavedra-Molina A. Cellular and mitochondrial effects of alcohol consumption. Int J Environ Res Public Health. 2010;7(12):4281-4304.

[120] Rubin E, et al. Alcohol and mitochondria. Alcohol Clin Exp Res. 2001;25(5 Suppl):34S-38S.

[121] Mutlu E, et al. Intestinal dysbiosis: a possible mechanism of alcohol-induced endotoxemia. World J Gastroenterol. 2009;15(11):1306-1310.

[122] Keshavarzian A, et al. Leaky gut in alcoholic cirrhosis. Am J Gastroenterol. 1999;94(1):200-207.

[123] Szabo G, Mandrekar P. Focus on: alcohol and the immune system. Alcohol Res Health. 2009;33(1-2):58-67.

[124] Lazzarini S, et al. Alcohol and lymphatic function. Lymphat Res Biol. 2017;15(2):130-138.

[125] Schlosser E. Fast Food Nation. Boston: Houghton Mifflin; 2001.

[126] Environmental Working Group. Natural vs. artificial flavors. EWG Food Scores Database; 2020.

[127] Chassaing B, et al. Dietary emulsifiers directly alter human microbiota composition and gene expression ex vivo and in vivo. Gut. 2022;71(1):68-76.

[128] Viennois E, et al. Dietary emulsifier-induced low-grade inflammation promotes colon carcinogenesis. Cancer Res. 2017;77(1):27-40.

[129] Johansson ME, et al. The inner of the two Muc2 mucin-dependent mucus layers in colon is devoid of bacteria. Proc Natl Acad Sci USA. 2008;105(39):15064-15069.

[130] Lanigan M, et al. Toxicology of food preservatives and their effects on mitochondria. Food Chem Toxicol. 2019;130:224-237.

[131] Lachenmeier DW, et al. Benzene in soft drinks. Mol Nutr Food Res. 2008;52(3):338-351.

[132] Piper PB. Yeast superoxide dismutase mutants reveal a pro-oxidant action of weak organic acid food preservatives. Free Radic Biol Med. 1999;27(11-12):1219-1227.

[133] Distilled Spirits Council of the United States. Annual Industry Review. 2022.

[134] Zelber-Sagi S, et al. Comparison of fatty liver index with noninvasive methods for steatosis detection. World J Gastroenterol. 2013;19(1):57-64.

[135] Pollan M. In Defense of Food: An Eater's Manifesto. New York: Penguin Press; 2008.

[136] Paddon-Jones D, et al. Protein and healthy aging. Am J Clin Nutr. 2015;101(6):1339S-1345S.

[137] Andersen CJ. Bioactive egg components and inflammation. Nutrients. 2015;7(9):7889-7913.

[138] Fuller NR, et al. Effect of a high-egg diet on cardiometabolic risk factors in people with type 2 diabetes. Am J Clin Nutr. 2018;107(6):921-931.

[139] Karsten HD, et al. Vitamins A, E and fatty acid composition of the eggs of caged hens and pastured hens. Renew Agric Food Syst. 2010;25(1):45-54.

[140] Sapkota M, et al. Arsenic resistance in Campylobacter and poultry antimicrobial use. Appl Environ Microbiol. 2006;72:4751-4757.

[141] Mozaffarian D, Rimm EB. Fish intake, contaminants, and human health. JAMA. 2006;296(15):1885-1899.

[142] Hites RA, et al. Global assessment of organic contaminants in farmed salmon. Science. 2004;303(5655):226-229.

[143] Daley CA, et al. A review of fatty acid profiles and antioxidant content in grass-fed and grain-fed beef. Nutr J. 2010;9:10.

[144] Micha R, et al. Unprocessed red and processed meats and risk of coronary artery disease. Circulation. 2010;121(21):2271-2283.

[145] Wiklund FW, et al. Muscle and fat quality in wild and reindeer. Meat Sci. 2000;55:157-164.

[146] Lebret A, et al. Influence of rearing conditions on performance and meat quality of pigs. Meat Sci. 2012;92:96-103.

[147] Ros E. Health benefits of nut consumption. Nutrients. 2010;2(7):652-682.

[148] Chen GC, et al. Nut consumption and risk of cardiovascular disease. Am J Clin Nutr. 2017;105(6):1462-1473.

[149] Ludwig DS, et al. Dietary carbohydrates: role of quality and quantity in chronic disease. BMJ. 2018;361:k2340.

[150] Tosh SM. Review of human studies investigating the post-prandial blood-glucose lowering ability of oat. Eur J Clin Nutr. 2013;67(4):310-317.

[151] El Khoury D, et al. Beta glucan: health benefits in obesity and metabolic syndrome. J Nutr Metab. 2012;2012:851362.

[152] Slavin J. Whole grains and human health. Nutr Res Rev. 2004;17(1):99-110.

[153] Vega-Galvez LE, et al. Nutrition facts and functional potential of quinoa. J Sci Food Agric. 2010;90(15):2541-2547.

[154] Tang G, et al. Golden Rice is an effective source of vitamin A. Am J Clin Nutr. 2012;96(3):658-664.

[155] Drewnowski A, Rehm CD. Vegetable cost metrics show potatoes and beans provide most nutrients per penny. PLoS One. 2013;8(5):e63277.

[156] Messina V. Nutritional and health benefits of dried beans. Am J Clin Nutr. 2014;100 Suppl 1:437S-442S.

[157] Mozaffarian D, et al. Components of a cardioprotective diet: new insights. Circulation. 2011;123(24):2870-2891.

[158] Jacques PF, Lichtenstein AH. Sources of dietary fiber and cardiovascular disease. Curr Atheroscler Rep. 2010;12(6):398-403.

[159] Higdon JV, et al. Cruciferous vegetables and human cancer risk. Pharmacol Res. 2007;55(3):224-236.

[160] Shapiro TA, et al. Human metabolism and excretion of cancer chemoprotective glucosinolates and isothiocyanates. Cancer Epidemiol Biomarkers Prev. 1998;7(12):1091-1100.

[161] Siervo M, et al. Inorganic nitrate and beetroot juice supplementation reduces blood pressure in adults. J Nutr. 2013;143(6):818-826.

[162] Liu RH. Health-promoting components of fruits and vegetables in the diet. Adv Nutr. 2013;4(3):384S-392S.

[163] Popkin BM, et al. Water, hydration, and health. Nutr Rev. 2010;68(8):439-458.

[164] Platel K, Srinivasan K. Digestive stimulant action of spices: a myth or reality? Indian J Med Res. 2004;119(5):167-179.

[165] Block E. Garlic and Other Alliums: The Lore and the Science. Cambridge: Royal Society of Chemistry; 2010.

[166] He FJ, et al. Increased consumption of fruit and vegetables is related to a reduced risk of coronary heart disease. J Hum Hypertens. 2007;21(9):717-728.

[167] Devore EE, et al. Dietary intakes of berries and flavonoids in relation to cognitive decline. Ann Neurol. 2012;72(1):135-143.

[168] Krikorian R, et al. Blueberry supplementation improves memory in older adults. J Agric Food Chem. 2010;58(7):3996-4000.

[169] Ross JA, Kasum CM. Dietary flavonoids: bioavailability, metabolic effects, and safety. Annu Rev Nutr. 2002;22:19-34.

[170] Howatson G, et al. Effect of tart cherry juice on melatonin levels and enhanced sleep quality. Eur J Nutr. 2012;51(8):909-916.

[171] Hyson DA. A comprehensive review of apples and apple components and their relationship to human health. Adv Nutr. 2011;2(5):408-420.

[172] Brat CI, et al. Daily polyphenol intake in France from fruit and vegetables. J Nutr. 2006;136(9):2368-2373.

[173] Calder PC. Functional roles of fatty acids and their effects on human health. JPEN. 2015;39(1 Suppl):18S-32S.

[174] Beauchamp GK, et al. Phytochemistry: ibuprofen-like activity in extra-virgin olive oil. Nature. 2005;437(7055):45-46.

[175] Estruch R, et al. Primary prevention of cardiovascular disease with a Mediterranean diet. N Engl J Med. 2018;378:e34.

[176] Wong PWC, et al. Avocado oil: Characteristics, properties, and applications. Molecules. 2019;24(11):2172.

[177] St-Onge MP, Bosarge A. Weight-loss diet that includes consumption of medium-chain triacylglycerol oil. Am J Clin Nutr. 2008;87(3):621-626.

[178] Nevin KG, Rajamohan T. Virgin coconut oil supplemented diet increases the antioxidant status in rats. Food Chem. 2006;99(2):260-266.

[179] Sharma S, et al. Ghee: Its Properties, Importance and Health Benefits. Lipid Technol. 2017;29(2):21-24.

[180] Jacobs DR Jr, Tapsell LC. Food, not nutrients, is the fundamental unit in nutrition. Nutr Rev. 2007;65(10):439-450.

[181] Popkin BM, et al. The nutrition transition: new trends in the global diet. Nutr Rev. 1999;57(2):31-37.

[182] Lustig RH. Metabolic syndrome and the American diet: the sad state of affairs. Clin Chem. 2008;54(4):661-662.

[183] Ludwig DS, Ebbeling CB. The carbohydrate-insulin model of obesity: beyond 'calories in, calories out'. JAMA Intern Med. 2018;178(8):1098-1103.

[184] Furman D, et al. Chronic inflammation in the etiology of disease across the life span. Nat Med. 2019;25(12):1822-1832.

[185] Fasano A. Leaky gut and autoimmune diseases. Clin Rev Allergy Immunol. 2012;42(1):71-78.

[186] Colberg SR, et al. Exercise and type 2 diabetes. Diabetes Care. 2010;33(12):e147-e167.

[187] Eckel RH, et al. 2013 AHA/ACC guideline on lifestyle management to reduce cardiovascular risk. Circulation. 2014;129(25 Suppl 2):S76-S99.

[188] Jacka FN, et al. Association of Western and traditional diets with depression and anxiety in women. Am J Psychiatry. 2010;167(3):305-311.

[189] St-Onge MP, et al. Fiber and saturated fat are associated with sleep arousals and slow wave sleep. J Clin Sleep Med. 2016;12(1):19-24.

[190] Deslypere JP. Obesity and cancer. Metabolism. 1995;44(9 Suppl 3):24-27.

[191] Monteiro CA, et al. Ultra-processed foods: what they are and how to identify them. Public Health Nutr. 2019;22(5):936-941.

[192] Nestle M. Food Politics: How the Food Industry Influences Nutrition and Health. Berkeley: University of California Press; 2013.

[193] Wansink B. Mindless Eating: Why We Eat More Than We Think. New York: Bantam Books; 2006.

[194] Hall KD, et al. Ultra-processed diets cause excess calorie intake and weight gain. Cell Metab. 2019;30(1):67-77.

[195] Academy of Nutrition and Dietetics. Position of the Academy: total diet approach to healthy eating. J Acad Nutr Diet. 2013;113(2):307-317.

[196] Mensink RP, et al. Effects of dietary fatty acids and carbohydrates on the ratio of serum total to HDL cholesterol. Am J Clin Nutr. 2003;77(5):1146-1155.

[197] Simopoulos AP. The importance of the omega-6/omega-3 fatty acid ratio in cardiovascular disease and other chronic diseases. Exp Biol Med. 2008;233(6):674-688.

[198] Lachat C, et al. Eating out of home and its association with dietary intake. Obes Rev. 2012;13(4):329-346.

[199] Bland JS. The Disease Delusion. New York: Harper Wave; 2014.

[200] Mozaffarian D, et al. Changes in diet and lifestyle and long-term weight gain in women and men. N Engl J Med. 2011;364(25):2392-2404.

[201] U.S. Department of Agriculture. Dietary Guidelines for Americans, 2020-2025. 9th ed. 2020.

[202] Estruch R, et al. Primary prevention of cardiovascular disease with a Mediterranean diet. N Engl J Med. 2013;368(14):1279-1290.

[203] Siri-Tarino PW, et al. Saturated fat, carbohydrate, and cardiovascular disease. Am J Clin Nutr. 2010;91(3):502-509.

[204] Hu FB, et al. Dietary fat intake and the risk of coronary heart disease in women. N Engl J Med. 1997;337(21):1491-1499.

[205] Lachat CJ, et al. Dietary intake during travel and its determinants. Asia Pac J Clin Nutr. 2008;17(3):444-451.

[206] Drewnowski A, Specter SE. Poverty and obesity: the role of energy density and energy costs. Am J Clin Nutr. 2004;79(1):6-16.

[207] Hollis JF, et al. Weight loss during the intensive intervention phase of the weight-loss maintenance trial. Am J Prev Med. 2008;35(2):118-126.

[208] Bowman SA, et al. Effects of fast-food consumption on energy intake and diet quality. Pediatrics. 2004;113(1):112-118.

[209] Roberto CA, et al. Patchy progress on obesity prevention. Lancet. 2015;385(9985):2400-2409.

[210] Powell LM, et al. Nutritional content of menu offerings across major US restaurant chains. Public Health Nutr. 2014;17(1):87-96.

[211] Wansink B, Sobal J. Mindless eating: the 200 daily food decisions we overlook. Environ Behav. 2007;39(1):106-123.

[212] Dunbar R. Breaking bread: the functions of social eating. Adaptive Human Behavior and Physiology. 2017;3:198-211.

[213] de Castro JM. Social facilitation of food intake by humans. Physiol Behav. 1990;47(6):1129-1135.

[214] Herman CP, et al. The social facilitation of eating. Appetite. 2015;86:61-65.

[215] Mann T. Secrets from the Eating Lab. New York: Harper Wave; 2015.

[216] Leidy HJ, et al. The effects of consuming frequent, higher protein meals on appetite and satiety. Obesity. 2011;19(4):818-824.

[217] Vartanian LR, et al. Effects of soft drink consumption on nutrition and health. Am J Public Health. 2007;97(4):667-675.

[218] Burger KS, Stice E. Variability in reward responsivity and obesity. Curr Drug Abuse Rev. 2011;4(3):182-189.

[219] Polivy J, Herman CP. Dieting and binging: a causal analysis. Am Psychol. 1985;40(2):193-201.

[220] Gilhooly CH, et al. Food cravings and energy regulation: the characteristics of craved foods. Int J Obes. 2007;31(12):1849-1858.

[221] Lieberman DE. The Story of the Human Body: Evolution, Health, and Disease. New York: Vintage; 2014.

[222] Wadden TA, et al. One-year weight losses in the Look AHEAD study. Obesity. 2009;17(4):713-722.

[223] Wing RR, Hill JO. Successful weight loss maintenance. Annu Rev Nutr. 2001;21:323-341.

[224] USDA Food Safety and Inspection Service. Safe food storage guidelines. 2023.

[225] Ford ES, et al. Healthy living is the best revenge. Arch Intern Med. 2009;169(15):1355-1362.

[226] Drewnowski A. Taste preferences and food intake. Annu Rev Nutr. 1997;17:237-253.

[227] Wansink B, et al. The office candy dish: proximity's influence on estimated and actual consumption. Int J Obes. 2006;30(5):871-875.

[228] Wardle J, et al. Evidence for a strong genetic influence on childhood adiposity. Am J Clin Nutr. 2008;87(2):398-404.

[229] Rozin P, et al. The ecology of eating: smaller portion sizes in France than in the United States. Psychol Sci. 2003;14(5):450-454.

[230] Matheson DM, et al. Children's food consumption during television viewing. Am J Clin Nutr. 2004;79(6):1088-1094.

[231] Boutelle KN, et al. How can parents and children eat together. J Am Diet Assoc. 2003;103(3):317-322.

[232] Neumark-Sztainer D, et al. Family meal patterns: associations with sociodemographic characteristics. J Am Diet Assoc. 2003;103(3):317-322.

[233] American Psychological Association. Stress and eating behaviors. 2022.

[234] Bureau of Labor Statistics. American Time Use Survey. 2023.

[235] Mozaffarian D, et al. Food compass is a nutrient profiling system using expanded characteristics for assessing healthfulness of foods. Nat Food. 2021;2:809-818.

[236] Gabel K, et al. Effects of 8-hour time restricted feeding on body weight and metabolic disease risk factors. Nutr Healthy Aging. 2018;4(4):345-353.

[237] Ornish D, et al. Intensive lifestyle changes for reversal of coronary heart disease. JAMA. 1998;280(23):2001-2007.

[238] Buettner D. The Blue Zones: Lessons for Living Longer from the People Who've Lived the Longest. Washington: National Geographic; 2012.

[239] Mann T, et al. Medicare's search for effective obesity treatments: diets are not the answer. Am Psychol. 2007;62(3):220-233.

[240] Dansinger ML, et al. Comparison of diets for weight loss and heart disease risk reduction. JAMA. 2005;293(1):43-53.

[241] Volkow ND, et al. Overlapping neuronal circuits in addiction and obesity. Philos Trans R Soc Lond B Biol Sci. 2008;363(1507):3191-3200.

[242] Wang GJ, et al. Brain dopamine and obesity. Lancet. 2001;357(9253):354-357.

[243] Johnson PM, Kenny PJ. Dopamine D2 receptors in addiction-like reward dysfunction. Nat Neurosci. 2010;13(5):635-641.

[244] Lustig RH. Fructose: it's 'alcohol without the buzz'. Adv Nutr. 2013;4(2):226-235.

[245] Ludwig DS. The glycemic index: physiological mechanisms. JAMA. 2002;287(18):2414-2423.

[246] Teff KL, et al. Dietary fructose reduces circulating insulin and leptin. J Clin Endocrinol Metab. 2004;89(6):2963-2972.

[247] Schwartz MW, et al. Central nervous system control of food intake. Nature. 2000;404(6778):661-671.

[248] Calder PC. Omega-3 fatty acids and inflammatory processes: evidence, mechanisms and relevance. Biochim Biophys Acta. 2015;1851(4):469-484.

[249] Foster JA, McVey Neufeld KA. Gut-brain axis: how the microbiome influences anxiety and depression. Trends Neurosci. 2013;36(5):305-312.

[250] Patterson E, et al. Intermittent fasting and human metabolic health. J Acad Nutr Diet. 2015;115(8):1203-1212.

[251] Longo VD, Panda S. Fasting, circadian rhythms, and time-restricted feeding in healthy lifespan. Cell Metab. 2016;23(6):1048-1059.

[252] Yanovski JA, et al. A prospective study of holiday weight gain. N Engl J Med. 2000;342(12):861-867.

[253] Yanovski JA. Trends in underweight and obesity. N Engl J Med. 2015;372(19):1862-1863.

[254] Vartanian LR, et al. Effects of soft drink consumption on nutrition and health. Am J Public Health. 2007;97(4):667-675.

[255] Gearhardt AN, et al. Neural correlates of food addiction. Arch Gen Psychiatry. 2011;68(8):808-816.

[256] Polivy J. Psychological consequences of food restriction. J Am Diet Assoc. 1996;96(6):589-592.

[257] Mischel W. The Marshmallow Test: Mastering Self-Control. New York: Little, Brown; 2014.

[258] Baumeister RF, Tierney J. Willpower: Rediscovering the Greatest Human Strength. New York: Penguin; 2011.

[259] Popkin BM, et al. Water, hydration, and health. Nutr Rev. 2010;68(8):439-458.

[260] Blumenthal JA, et al. Exercise and pharmacotherapy in the treatment of major depressive disorder. Psychosom Med. 2007;69(7):587-596.

[261] Stevenson AC, et al. Taste perception changes following weight loss or gain: a systematic review. Appetite. 2019;138:44-50.

[262] Wise M, et al. Reduced food cue reactivity after eating in the absence of hunger. Appetite. 2015;95:103-107.

[263] Brunstrom JM. The control of meal size in human subjects. Proc Nutr Soc. 2011;70(2):155-161.

[264] Wardle J, Gibson JA. Impact of stress on diet: processes and implications. In: Stansfeld S, Marmot M, eds. Stress and the Heart. London: BMJ Books; 2002.

[265] Schvey NA, et al. The stress-eating paradox. Int J Eat Disord. 2016;49(3):327-330.

[266] Brownell KD. Dieting and the search for the perfect body. Behav Ther. 1991;22(1):1-12.

[267] Gearhardt AN, et al. Preliminary validation of the Yale Food Addiction Scale. Appetite. 2009;52(2):430-436.

[268] Sampson HA. Food allergy: accurately identifying clinical reactivity. Allergy. 2005;60 Suppl 79:19-24.

[269] Muraro A, et al. EAACI Food Allergy and Anaphylaxis Guidelines: diagnosis and management. Allergy. 2014;69(8):1008-1025.

[270] Sicherer SH, Sampson HA. Food allergy: epidemiology, pathogenesis, diagnosis, and treatment. J Allergy Clin Immunol. 2014;133(2):291-307.

[271] Boyce JA, et al. Guidelines for the diagnosis and management of food allergy in the United States. J Allergy Clin Immunol. 2010;126(6 Suppl):S1-S58.

[272] Sampson HA, et al. Fatal and near-fatal anaphylactic reactions to food in children and adolescents. N Engl J Med. 1992;327(6):380-384.

[273] Burks AW, et al. ICON: food allergy. J Allergy Clin Immunol. 2012;129(4):906-920.

[274] Gupta RS, et al. Prevalence and severity of food allergies among US adults. JAMA Netw Open. 2019;2(1):e185630.

[275] Mullin GE, et al. Testing for food reactions: the good, the bad, and the ugly. Nutr Clin Pract. 2010;25(2):192-198.

[276] Zopf Y, et al. The differential diagnosis of food intolerance. Dtsch Arztebl Int. 2009;106(21):359-369.

[277] Swagerty DL Jr, et al. Lactose intolerance. Am Fam Physician. 2002;65(9):1845-1850.

[278] Maintz L, Novak N. Histamine and histamine intolerance. Am J Clin Nutr. 2007;85(5):1185-1196.

[279] Gibson PR, Shepherd SJ. Evidence-based dietary management of functional gastrointestinal symptoms. J Gastroenterol Hepatol. 2010;25(2):252-258.

[280] Mullin GE, et al. Food sensitivity testing. Integr Med. 2016;15(4):32-37.

[281] Vojdani A, et al. A review of food allergy testing: promise and pitfalls. Altern Ther Health Med. 2011;17(1):34-41.

[282] Vojdani A. For the assessment of intestinal permeability, size matters. Altern Ther Health Med. 2013;19(1):12-24.

[283] Arroyave Hernandez CM, et al. Food allergy mediated by IgG antibodies associated with migraine. Rev Alerg Mex. 2007;54(5):162-168.

[284] Institute for Functional Medicine. Elimination diet comprehensive guide. 2019.

[285] Skypala I, et al. Sensitivity to food additives, vaso-active amines and salicylates. Clin Transl Allergy. 2015;5:34.

[286] Sicherer SH. Clinical implications of cross-reactive food allergens. J Allergy Clin Immunol. 2001;108(6):881-890.

[287] Katz J. Managing diet in GI disease. Gastroenterol Clin North Am. 2007;36(2):361-381.

[288] Pizzorno J. Toxins in the gut and intestinal permeability. Integr Med. 2014;13(6):8-11.

[289] Consumer Reports. Food sensitivity testing: what you need to know. 2022.

[290] USDA Food Safety and Inspection Service. Meat and poultry labeling terms. 2022.

[291] Environmental Working Group. Meat Eater's Guide to Climate Change and Health. 2011.

[292] Alfaia CM, et al. Effect of the feeding system on intramuscular fatty acids. Meat Sci. 2009;114(3):939-946.

[293] Consumer Reports. How to buy safer, more nutritious eggs. 2022.

[294] Mozaffarian D, et al. Dietary and policy priorities to reduce the global crises of obesity and diabetes. Health Aff. 2012;31(1):166-174.

[295] Daley CA, et al. A review of fatty acid profiles and antioxidant content in grass-fed and grain-fed beef. Nutr J. 2010;9:10.

[296] Hites RA, et al. Global assessment of organic contaminants in farmed salmon. Science. 2004;303(5655):226-229.

[297] Carpenter DO, et al. Health risks of persistent organic pollutants from long-range atmospheric transport. Environ Health Perspect. 2005;113(5):552-556.

[298] Karsten HD, et al. Vitamins A, E and fatty acid composition of eggs from caged hens and pastured hens. Renew Agric Food Syst. 2010;25(1):45-54.

[299] Poulain M, et al. Identification of a geographic area characterized by extreme longevity in the Sardinia island. Exp Gerontol. 2004;39(9):1423-1429.

[300] Institute of Medicine. Dietary Reference Intakes for Energy, Carbohydrate, Fiber, Fat, Fatty Acids, Cholesterol, Protein, and Amino Acids. Washington: National Academies Press; 2005.

[301] Naviaux RK. Metabolic features of the cell danger response. Mitochondrion. 2014;16:7-17.

www.ingramcontent.com/pod-product-compliance
Lightning Source LLC
Chambersburg PA
CBHW071431230926
51846CB00001B/185
* 9 7 8 1 9 7 1 4 4 9 0 3 6 *